ABOUT THIS BOOK

The inspiration for this book came after many years of fellow Moms asking me questions about how I feed my kids. Knowing that I was a Registered Dietitian *and* a mother of 3 boys, Moms would ask me food-related questions while watching our kids' play baseball and soccer or while standing outside of school waiting for the bell to ring.

Among the many, many conversations, some of the most common questions were:

> "Do you allow your kids to eat chips?"
> "What do you think of sports drinks?"
> "How often do your kids eat Fast Food?"

The short answers are occasionally; not much; and about once every 6 months. The longer, more useful answers you'll find in this book.

In the midst of one of these conversations, I thought, "I wonder what other Registered Dietitians do? Would their answers be the same as mine?" It occurred to me that the ideas and strategies I use might be different than what other Nutrition Experts have found useful, and wouldn't it be great to share all of these ideas with Moms everywhere, not just in my community!

So I embarked on surveying Registered Dietitians who willingly and graciously answered all of my questions. Over 400 Nutrition Experts provided input to help make this book a comprehensive "Go-To" guide for Moms like you.

My hope for you is that after reading this book, you have answers to your questions and simple, practical strategies that help you provide healthier choices to your child.

Here's to your healthy, thriving child!

Jill West, RD

The information contained in this book is designed to provide general nutrition guidelines for children with no food allergies or medical conditions that may require specialized dietary recommendations.

In addition, this book is not intended to take the place of a doctor's or health care provider's recommendations, and should not be construed as a substitute for professional medical advice or care. Please contact your doctor for specific medical and nutrition-related questions, diagnoses, care, and recommendations.

Published by JD West Consulting, Inc.
PO Box 6636
Moraga, CA 94570

ISBN 13 : 978-0-9893712-0-9

Illustration: Cathy Boylan-Swan *www.boylanstudios.net*
Cover Design / Book Layout: Mike Swan   *www.bc-creative.com*

DEDICATION

To my wonderful boys, Jonathan, Michael and Jason.
You are the joy of my life!

To my husband, Dan, for always believing in me.

ACKNOWLEDGEMENTS

Writing a book can be deeply rewarding, but at times a very lonely and isolating experience. But thanks to my supportive husband and my eternally optimistic 3 boys, I would end the day knowing I could and would complete the next chapter and finally the entire book. As Jason says, "Mom, you gotta believe!" Thank you so much for your support!

I must also thank my friend and colleague, Dianne Hyson, Ph.D., M.S., R.D., for enthusiastically supporting my book idea; helping me create the survey that became the foundation of this book; and editing the book as it neared completion.

Thank you to all the Registered Dietitians who willingly and enthusiastically completed the survey. Your ideas, tips and strategies are a great contribution to this book.

Thank you to my dedicated reviewers who generously gave their time, providing great suggestions and feedback. Your input and support has been so valuable and appreciated!

Thank you to Cathy Boylan-Swan, illustrator, for your patience and great work and to Mike Swan, book and website designer, for working tirelessly to get the content, book cover and website just right.

Finally, I am deeply indebted to Kevin O'Brien. Without him, this book would not have come to fruition. His knowledge, experience and enthusiasm made my dream of writing a book come true.

I am eternally grateful to you all!

Jill

A Word About Food Allergies...

Of the many ideas and suggestions presented in this book, one topic not covered is Food Allergies and Intolerances, which is complicated enough to deserve its own book.

It's an area that's getting much more attention and definitely requires input from medical professionals, such as doctors and registered dietitians, who specialize in this field.

If your child has symptoms such as headaches, skin irritations (rashes, hives, eczema) or gastrointestinal symptoms (nausea, vomiting, diarrhea) that are on-going and not explained by a virus or other illness, you should consider meeting with a specialist and having further testing done.

Some examples of allergy testing include the RAST test, which is a skin test or the ALCAT test which is a simple blood test. You can learn more about the ALCAT test by going to the website: www.alcat.com.

Specialists can combine these tests with a thorough medical history and food diary analysis to make a diagnosis and ensure that your child grows and thrives with a diet that is balanced, despite having to eliminate certain foods.

If you want to explore food allergies in more detail, a really great, reliable resource can be found at this website:

www.nal.usda.gov/fnic/pubs/bibs/allegy.pdf

• • •

TABLE OF CONTENTS

CHAPTER 1

INTRODUCTION

"Moms Have So Much Influence Over The Health Of Their Kids"

– Jill West

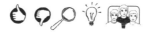

Introduction :

I know raising a healthy child is important to you because you're reading these words. Being a Mom myself, I know you're busy, have many responsibilities, and your time is precious. Reading a book doesn't always make the priority list. So I've designed this book as a "Go-To" guide that allows you to read it cover to cover or skip around, choosing specific chapters that are most important to you and your family.

But there's still the question of "What's in it for you?" Why read this book? Well, if your child is overweight the reasons are many. Overweight & obese kids and adolescents are at risk for many health problems, both as kids and as adults. Do you really want your child to have high blood pressure or high cholesterol as a teenager? What about Type 2 Diabetes? Unfortunately, that's the reality for your child if he or she is overweight.

Imagine your child at school being bullied and called names because of his weight. If you were ever bullied in school you know how much it affects your life. One recent study found that being overweight increased the risk of being bullied by 63%! Teasing and bullying are unacceptable for sure and many parents feel helpless when it comes to bullying. One really great way you can make a difference and support your child is to provide healthy foods and help them be active every day.

The toll of excess weight is both physical and emotional. Picture your child playing at recess and not being able to run and keep up with the other kids because her weight slows her down. Kids in this situation are less likely to play active games, are more likely to be teased and have more difficulty forming friendships, all contributing to low self-esteem.

You might be thinking why read this book if your child isn't overweight? Imagine your child sitting at school fidgeting in his chair or staring off into space while the teacher is teaching math. Did he have a high-sugar breakfast? What did he eat for lunch? You can make a huge difference in your child's attention span and academic performance by making healthy eating a priority.

For example, eating a healthy breakfast is associated with improved daily attendance, better test scores and greater class participation. Poor nutrition is linked to more frequent colds and flu, causing more days missed from school. By insisting your child makes healthy choices at breakfast and lunch, you're doing your job as a parent to ensure your child's success at school.

Finally, this book is a must read for all parents, but especially Moms. Why? Because Moms are the "gatekeepers" when it comes to food for the family. I know Dads are more involved in grocery shopping and cooking and other caretakers can also fill the role of Moms when it comes to food, but women continue to do the majority of the grocery shopping and have the most influence on food decisions. Managing the grocery list, planning and preparing meals and deciding which restaurants your family goes to is an incredibly important job. **You have so much influence over the health of your child. Seize the opportunity now!**

 Woven throughout the book are the experiences, strategies and advice of over 400 Registered Dietitians that I surveyed.

These Nutrition Experts are Moms with busy lives just like you. And despite the barrage of heavily processed, high fat, high sugar foods in our world, they've found ways to consistently provide healthy food to their kids. You can too! This book will give you strategies that work in the real world. Whether you're a working Mom or a stay-at-home Mom, you'll find dozens of ideas you can use every day that help you serve healthy choices without spending all day in the kitchen.

More specifically, you'll get:
  Practical Tips for quick, healthy meals and snacks.
  Real **Strategies** to get your kids to eat healthy foods.
  Simple Solutions for lowering the sugar, fat and "empty calories" your kids eat.

My approach when working with families is to encourage realistic strategies that are achievable and sustainable for the long-term. My philosophy is :

Small changes lead to big success!

I've used this philosophy in this book and offer many ideas, tips and strategies that are simple and doable for busy parents. You can choose which healthy strategies you want to try with your family. Over time these small, healthy changes become healthy habits that you and your kids can continue for a lifetime.

What To Expect :

Throughout the book I use the terms Registered Dietitian and Nutrition Experts interchangeably and am referring to nutrition professionals who have received a nutrition-related Bachelor's or Master's degree and advanced training in nutrition, along with passing a national registration exam.

There are a few topics I decided not to focus on in this book, including details about organic foods, calorie and fat requirements, and artificial sweeteners. I will briefly address each of these topics.

Organic Foods
Although I believe organic foods are a great choice, what's most important is that kids are eating fruits and vegetables whether they are organic or not. I'm concerned that people who can't afford organic produce will ultimately eat less fruits and vegetables because they think the non-organic choices are too harmful to eat, and that's not true. I'm certainly in favor of ingesting as little pesticides as possible, but research shows the benefits of eating fruits and vegetables outweighs the risk of pesticide exposure. The amount of pesticides we get from foods grown in this country is very small and the harmful effects of NOT EATING produce is much greater. This is what I suggest:
- Eat fruits and vegetables that are in season, mostly from the U.S. and as local as possible.
- If you are concerned about pesticides, but can't afford all organic produce, check the list on page 235 that shows which fruits and vegetables are most important to choose organic and which produce is less important to buy organic. You can also go to this website for more information: http://www.ewg.org/foodnews/summary

Calories and Fat

I haven't included information about the calorie and fat requirements for kids for the following reasons:

#1 : The calorie needs for children can vary significantly based on their activity levels, age and genetics. **What's most important is providing your child with nutrient-rich calories instead of "empty" calories.** I'll talk about empty calories in more detail throughout the book. If you're concerned about specific calorie or nutrient needs for your child, I recommend you meet with a registered dietitian.

#2 : Rather than focusing on how many calories your child needs for the whole day, I provide calorie and fat information in the Best Picks, Worst Picks and "Go-To" Guide as a reference point to help you understand what is too many calories or too much unhealthy saturated fat for an individual serving. Fat is very important in a child's diet and should not be restricted, but it should come from healthy sources. I've included a list of healthy fats on page 236.

Artificial Sweeteners

I believe that minimizing the amount of artificial sweeteners a child gets is important, but there are situations where I think they are a reasonable choice in moderation. For example, if your child is overweight or has Diabetes and controlling calories and/or sugar are important, then choosing foods that have artificial sweetener can be useful and appropriate. I believe this is an individual decision, but there is no research showing that small amounts of artificial sweetener are harmful. Like everything else, it's all about moderation.

Each chapter consists of 4 components. First, there's the "meat" of the chapter with facts, figures and important nutrition information for you to know. Next, you'll find tips, strategies, kid-approved recipes and quick-reference lists of foods to choose (Best Picks) and foods to avoid (Worst Picks).

Near the end of each chapter you'll always find a summary that I call *The Bottom Line*, to highlight the most important "take home" message. Finally, you'll have an opportunity to set *Your Game Plan*, or what you plan to do differently to improve what your kids are eating regularly.

An Easy 4-Step Process :

As you read a chapter there's a 4-step process that will help you start making changes right away. Here's how easy it's going to be:

STEP 1 :
Read the chapter.

STEP 2 :
Based on what you learned, think about what changes are needed for your kids to be healthier.

STEP 3 :
In the section called Your Game Plan, decide what change or changes are "a good place to start" for you and your family.

STEP 4 :
Consistently repeat Your Game Plan while you read another chapter.

Let me explain a little more about Steps 3 & 4. What I mean by *"a good place to start"* is what change or changes are realistic for your family. I encourage you to always make the easiest changes first. Why? Because we all like positive results and to feel successful! By having some early "wins", you can build on that success and make bigger or additional changes as time goes on.

Always remember that ***Change is a Process***. I've found that trying to change too much, too quickly usually backfires, and, ultimately, little or no progress is made. Making realistic changes that you can follow through on consistently is far better than grand plans to overhaul all your kids' food choices with everyone kicking and screaming. The overhaul won't be maintainable, causes a lot of stress and leads to everyone giving up.

The reason I've included ***Your Game Plan*** is to help you *take action* right away, after reading the chapter. By writing down 2 or 3 "Action Steps", you're beginning the process of change. Make your Action Steps specific and realistic so that you and your kids can repeat them for several days, weeks and months. Your Action Steps are new *behaviors*. Repetition of these new behaviors is the key to creating new healthy *habits*.

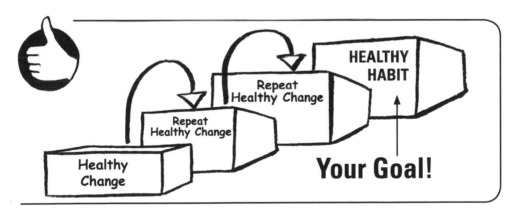

For example, after reading the chapter about beverages you decide you want to decrease the amount of juice and Gatorade your kids drink. That's a great plan, but it needs to be more specific. So your plan might be to serve juice 2 days/week and Gatorade no more than once/week. Now your plan is specific and you can track your progress because you know how many days you're aiming for. You also need to ask yourself, "Is this plan realistic?" If your kids are drinking juice and Gatorade daily, then you might need to start a little slower or choose one drink to decrease. Then you can work on decreasing the other sweet drink in a month or so.

Make Your Game Plan Work :

After you set *Your Game Plan*, you'll want to answer the question, "What will help my Game Plan work?" It's essential to have support and strategies in place in order for *Your Game Plan* to work. If you just *say* you're going to make a change, it's not going to happen. But if you have strategies in place that help you take action, then you're much more likely to have success.

So let's go back to the previous example. You decide *Your Game Plan* is to decrease the juice your kids drink to 2 days/week. Ok, the next step is to think about what strategies could help this goal happen.

Some examples of strategies are :

1. I will talk to my kids about decreasing juice and why we're doing it.

2. I will serve juice on Tuesdays and Fridays at breakfast.

3. I will buy a smaller carton of juice.

There are many strategies besides these examples that could support your plan. The main idea is to decide what you can do to help *Your Game Plan* succeed.

Being very specific about your plan and having strategies or support in place, increases the odds that you'll **start** a new behavior and **be successful** with the change you set out to make.

In working with families, I've found that it takes 6 to 12 months before new, healthy behaviors are truly habits. So be patient with yourself, your kids and the process as you make healthy changes.

It's also important to know that "backsliding" can be a normal part of the process of changing old habits and routines. It will take time, repetition and sometimes starting over a few times before the new, healthier ways become what I call "the no-brainer", which are the healthy things you do, buy and prepare regularly, without thinking much about it.

One More Thing…Change can be difficult for both kids and adults. You can expect some resistance from your kids and possibly even your spouse, as you make changes in the foods you buy, where you eat out or the meals you make at home. With time, though, the resistance decreases as the new ways become the routine.

During moments of resistance, keep in mind, you're providing a gift for a lifetime by helping your kids learn how to eat and be healthy!

Making healthy eating a priority *will* make a difference in your child's health, growth and learning. Let this book guide you through the high fat, high sugar, heavily processed world we live in and *still* raise healthy, thriving kids!

CHAPTER 2

BREAKFAST

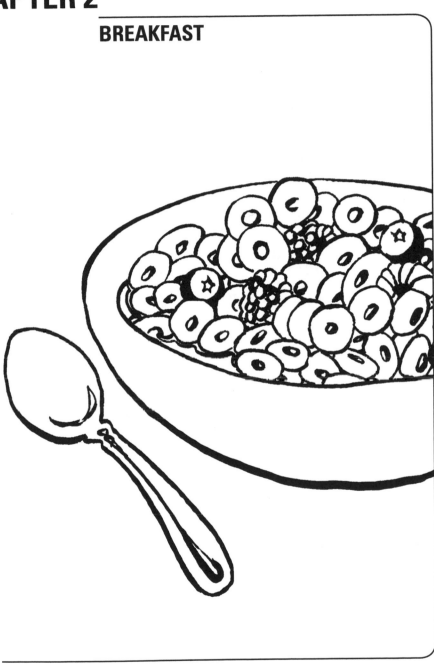

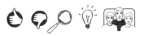

Breakfast . . .
A "Must-Have" Meal!

DID YOU KNOW . . .
As many as 37% of American kids and young adults skip breakfast?

Providing breakfast for your child is one of the most important things you can do as a parent. Why? Kids who eat breakfast have longer attention spans, better memory and higher test scores at school.

Not only that, kids who eat breakfast have better moods, better overall nutrition and healthier weights than those who skip breakfast regularly. By making sure your child eats breakfast, you're giving them a GIFT! The gift of good health and success in school.

As kids get older, eating breakfast declines by as much as 25%

Research shows a significant decline in breakfast intake in the 12 - 19 year-old group. So just as the demands of school begin to increase, breakfast decreases, putting tweens and teens at greater risk of poor concentration, poor attention and potentially lower test scores.

The solution?
Insist your child
eats breakfast daily!

Just like your car and cell phone, your child needs refueling and recharging. Breakfast is designed to "break your fast" from the 8 to 12 hours that have passed since the last meal or snack the night before.

Foods containing carbohydrate (fruits, bread products, cereals) give the body energy. Most importantly, your brain relies on carbohydrate for fuel and to function at its best. As a parent, I want to send my kids off to school well fueled, so they are ready to concentrate and learn at their best. I bet you do too.

By combining protein with carbohydrate at breakfast, your child will stay full longer and get valuable nutrients.

For example, milk, nuts, peanut butter, yogurt, cottage cheese, string cheese, eggs, beans, vegetarian sausage or tofu are all healthy protein choices for breakfast. When you combine one of these protein choices with a carbohydrate choice, the breakfast meal is more complete.

I've learned that once my child gets hungry, food is the only thing he can focus on until that belly gets filled again - so I want him satisfied at school so he's focused on learning, not on food.

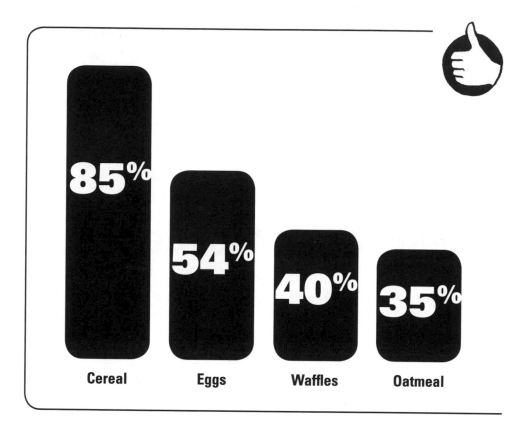

The #1 breakfast Registered Dietitians feed their kids is . . .

Ready-To-Eat Cereal with Non-Fat or 1% Milk

Ready-to-eat cereals are simple, fast and convenient

The most popular cereal cited by Nutrition Experts : Cheerios

Why? Nutritionally, Cheerios is a low sugar, ready-to-eat cereal, that also has fiber. *NOTE : Regular and Multi-Grain Cheerios are the two low-sugar varieties.*

Cheerios are also fortified with several vitamins and minerals, including iron. It's an excellent choice for all ages (toddlers through adults), and when combined with milk and fruit, it makes a quick, well-balanced meal to start the day.

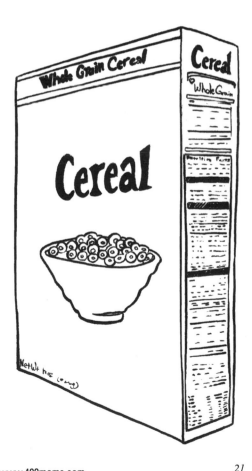

Cheerios
The Most Popular
CEREAL
Registered Dietitians
Feed Their Kids

When choosing cereals, read the label carefully . . .

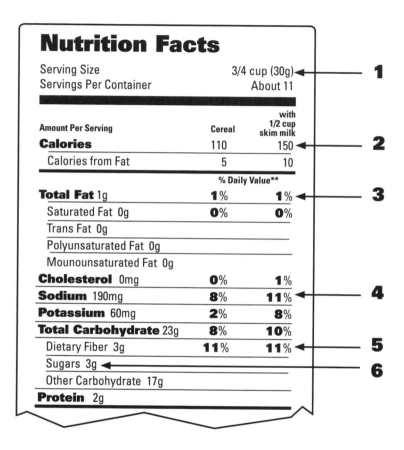

Nutrition Facts

Serving Size		3/4 cup (30g) ◄ — **1**
Servings Per Container		About 11

Amount Per Serving	Cereal	with 1/2 cup skim milk
Calories	110	150 ◄ — **2**
Calories from Fat	5	10

	% Daily Value**	
Total Fat 1g	**1**%	**1**% ◄ — **3**
Saturated Fat 0g	**0**%	**0**%
Trans Fat 0g		
Polyunsaturated Fat 0g		
Mounounsaturated Fat 0g		
Cholesterol 0mg	**0**%	**1**%
Sodium 190mg	**8**%	**11**% ◄ — **4**
Potassium 60mg	**2**%	**8**%
Total Carbohydrate 23g	**8**%	**10**%
Dietary Fiber 3g	**11**%	**11**% ◄ — **5**
Sugars 3g ◄ — **6**		
Other Carbohydrate 17g		
Protein 2g		

What to look for on a cereal label :

1. SERVING SIZE – The serving listed is not always the serving we eat, so knowing how much cereal you pour into the bowl is very important for knowing how many calories and other nutrients your child is actually getting. Pour the serving size listed on the cereal box into a measuring cup. Now pour it into the bowl your child uses to see how it fills the bowl. Now you know what one serving looks like.

2. CALORIES – are listed for a single serving. If your child eats more than one serving, his calorie intake will be greater than what is listed on the label.

3. TOTAL FAT – Most cereals are low in fat, which helps make them a healthy choice. If the cereal contains nuts, the fat may be higher than other cereals, but is still a healthy choice since nuts are a healthy source of fat.

4. SODIUM – Look for cereals with less than 250 mg sodium per serving. Grains are naturally low in sodium, so the goal is to keep them that way! In general the more a food is processed, the higher the sodium content. For example, ½ cup of plain rolled oats (makes 1 cup cooked oatmeal) has **0 mg sodium**, but a ready-to-eat cold cereal made from oats (which is more processed) now has **185-250mg sodium.** Although the sodium in this example is in the healthy range, eating too many processed foods leads to eating too much sodium, which can increase blood pressure and increase the risk of heart attack, stroke, congestive heart failure and kidney disease.

5. FIBER - 3 grams of fiber per serving is defined as a "good source" of fiber. Serve cereals with at least 3 grams of fiber most of the time. If you have a hard time getting your child to eat high fiber cereals, mix a high fiber cereal with her favorite cereal to boost the fiber and keep it tasty.

6. SUGAR – for cereals, less than 6 grams of sugar per serving is considered low in sugar; however, if there's dried fruit in the cereal, the grams of natural sugar from fruit will also be included here. Unfortunately, there isn't a way to determine how much of the sugar is added to the cereal and how much is from fruit. One strategy is to read the ingredient list and choose cereals with as few sugar sources as possible. Below is a list of types of sugar that you might find on the ingredient list:

corn syrup	*confectioner's sugar*	*corn syrup solids*
rice syrup	*invert sugar*	*molasses*
malt syrup	*brown sugar*	*honey*
cane syrup	*beet sugar*	*fructose*
maple syrup	*turbinado sugar*	*glucose*
cane sugar	*high fructose corn syrup*	

CEREAL FACTS

Reading the Nutrition Facts label is the most accurate way to make sure you're getting what you think you're getting. The 2 most important nutrients to focus on are:

SUGAR : 6 grams or less
FIBER : 3 grams or more

Next, read the ingredient list looking for whole grains in the top 3 ingredients. Examples of whole grains would be
* *whole wheat flour*   * *whole oat flour*
* *rolled oats*   * *brown rice flour*

Buyer Beware: ingredients listed as "wheat flour" and "enriched wheat flour" are really processed white flour. Ingredients are listed in order by weight, so the first two or three ingredients make up the majority of what's in the cereal. By choosing cereals that have "whole" grains your child gets valuable fiber and vitamins.

I also suggest you count up how many types of sugar are listed in the ingredient list because when they're all combined, sugar might actually be higher on the ingredient list than it appears.

For example, Kellogg's Cracklin' Oat Bran sounds like it should be healthy since it has oat bran in it, but looking carefully at the ingredient list you'll see that it not only contains brown sugar, but also corn syrup, sugar, and malt syrup. When all of these are added together, sugar becomes a main ingredient.

**Cereal is a heavily advertised product
and aggressively marketed to children.**

**Unfortunately, most of these cereals are filled with sugar,
as much as 3 to 4 teaspoons of sugar per serving!**

HIGH-SUGAR Cereals

An interesting study... Kids aged 5 to 12 years old were randomly assigned to choose one of three low-sugar cereals or one of three high-sugar cereals. The kids also had unlimited access to low fat milk, orange juice, bananas, strawberries and packets of sugar.

There were some very interesting results from this study:

- 54% of children who got low-sugar cereal **added fruit on top**, compared to only 8% of kids who got high-sugar cereal.

- Kids who had high-sugar cereal ate **twice as much added sugar**, even when the researchers added in the sugar from sugar packets the kids used on their low-sugar cereal.

- Kids who had high-sugar cereal **ate almost double** the amount of cereal compared to kids having low-sugar cereal.

What does all this mean?
By serving low sugar cereals, your child is much more likely to eat fruit at breakfast and get less total sugar, even if they add some sugar to their cereal. That's a winning combination!

Many of us go through the grocery store on "auto-pilot" plunking boxes into our grocery cart, choosing products out of habit or to stop a whining child. But when you stop to look at what is in your grocery cart and the potentially harmful effects of a high sugar diet, it's time to rethink your choices.

Kids who regularly eat foods high in sugar are less likely to get the quality nutrients their growing bodies need. High sugar foods are "empty calories", meaning they have very few nutrients and take the place of healthy, whole foods, which are loaded with vitamins, minerals and phytochemicals that keep us healthy.

IMPORTANT ... High sugar foods are "calorie dense", or high in calories for a small portion. Eating calorie dense foods regularly can lead to excessive weight gain in kids and adults. Although it's thought that sugar intake does not directly cause diabetes, when high sugar intake leads to weight gain, then the risk of diabetes, heart disease and high blood pressure increases in kids, just like it does in adults. Currently in the United States, all three of these diseases are on a dramatic rise in our kids.

 DID YOU KNOW ... Current health trends show that for the first time in history our children are expected to have shorter lives than their parents! *They are expected to live 2 to 5 years less because of obesity and the medical problems related to obesity.*

Jill's Worst Picks :
Worst Cereal Choices

Manufacturer	BRAND	Grams of Sugar	% of Calories from Sugar
Kellogg's	Honey Smacks	15	60 %
Quaker	Cap'n Crunch	12	44 %
Kellogg's	Cocoa Krispies	12	40 %
Quaker	Cap'n Crunch Crunch Berries	11	44 %
Kellogg's	Frosted Flakes	11	40 %
General Mills	Cocoa Puffs	10	40 %
General Mills	Lucky Charms	10	37 %
General Mills	Reese's Puffs	10	33 %
Post	Cocoa Pebbles	10	33 %
General Mills	Golden Grahams	10	33 %
Kellogg's	Apple Jacks	9	48 %
Kellogg's	Fruit Loops	9	44 %
Post	Fruity Pebbles	9	33 %
General Mills	Cookie Crisp	9	36 %
General Mills	Cinnamon Toast Crunch	9	28 %

Note the shocking amount of sugar that's in many popular cereals . . .

When reading the Nutrition Facts labels for these cereals you'll notice the serving size varies from ¾ cup to 1 cup. In order to accurately compare the sugar content between cereals, I used a consistent **serving size of ¾ cup** for all cereals and calculated the sugar content based on a ¾ cup serving. Keep in mind that most of us don't eat ¾ cup of cereal. **Your child could easily be eating 2 or 3 times this amount and, therefore, eating double or triple the amount of sugar listed.**

How much sugar is in each gram?

Approximately 4 grams of sugar is equal to one teaspoon. So if your child eats 1-1/2 cups of Quaker Cap'n Crunch, she is eating 24 grams of sugar, which equals **6 teaspoons of sugar!**

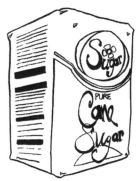

Jill's Best Picks :
Best Low-Sugar Cereals

Manufacturer	BRAND	Grams of Sugar	% of Calories from Sugar
Quaker	Oatmeal (plain)	1	3 %
General Mills	Cheerios	1	4 %
Trader Joe's	O's	1	4 %
General Mills	Rice Chex	1.5	8 %
General Mills	Corn Chex	2	10 %
General Mills	Kix	2	11 %
Kellogg's	Corn Flakes	2	12 %
Kellogg's	Rice Krispies	2.5	12 %
Kellogg's	Special K (original)	3	13 %
Kellogg's	Crispix	3	14 %
Kellogg's	Product-19	3	14 %
Fiber One	Honey Clusters	4.5	15 %
Kashi	Go Lean	4.5	17 %
General Mills	Multi-Grain Cheerios	4.5	22 %
General Mills	Wheat Chex	5	12 %
Kashi	Autumn Wheat	5	16 %
Barbara's Bakery	Shredded Spoonfuls	5	17 %
Kashi	Heart To Heart	5	17 %
General Mills	TOTAL	5	20 %
Barbara's Bakery	Puffins	5	22 %

It's more important to check the grams of sugar, not the % of sugar.

You may have noticed that the % of calories from sugar can be different even when the grams of sugar are the same. This results from a difference in calories per serving for a given cereal. For example, if a cereal has 6 grams of sugar and a serving is 140 calories, the % of calories from sugar is 17%. But if a cereal has 6 grams of sugar and 90 calories per serving, the % of calories from sugar is 27%.

What About Fiber?

Although a cereal may be low in sugar, it may not meet the criteria for an "ideal" cereal if it's low in fiber. (Ideal cereals have $\leq$ 6 grams of sugar and $\geq$3 grams of fiber). On the other hand, there are some cereals that are high in fiber, but also higher in sugar.

So what's a Mom to do? In the next table I list what I think are the best cereals because they are both low in sugar and have fiber. The cereals are listed from highest to lowest in fiber to help you quickly identify which cereals have the most fiber (at the top of the list). I've included a few cereals that are slightly higher in sugar or slightly lower in fiber than the "ideal", but felt they were worth including because nutritionally they are a healthy choice and cereals kids will eat. These cereals are a great way for your child to start the day or to have as an afterschool snack. I highly recommend these cereals.

Jill's Best Picks :
Best High Fiber/Low Sugar Cereals

Manufacturer	BRAND	Grams of Fiber	Grams of Sugar
Kashi	**Go Lean**	**10**	**6**
General Mills	**Wheat Chex**	**6**	**5**
Barbara's Bakery	**Puffins** (original, honey rice or peanut butter)	**5**	**5**
Quaker	**Oatmeal (plain)**	**4**	**1**
Barbara's Bakery	**Shredded Spoonfuls**	**4**	**5**
Kashi	**Autumn Wheat**	**3**	**5**
General Mills	**Cheerios**	**3**	**1**
Trader Joe's	**O's**	**3**	**1**
General Mills	**Kix**	**3**	**3**
General Mills	**Total**	**3**	**5**
General Mills	**Multi-Grain Cheerios**	**3**	**6**
Quaker	**Whole Hearts**	**3**	**6**
Bear Naked	**Granola**	**2**	**6**
Post	**Honey Bunches of Oats**	**2**	**6**
Quaker	**Life**	**2**	**6**

The goal is to strike a balance: Purchase low sugar cereals with as much fiber as possible, while keeping variety and choices your child will eat.

EGGS ...
The 2nd most common breakfast
Nutrition Experts feed their kids

Although eggs take a bit longer to prepare, scrambled eggs & whole wheat toast is a common combination Nutrition Experts serve. Eggs & toast can be made in 5 minutes and provide a healthy combination of carbohydrate and protein to boost energy and stave off hunger until lunchtime. By adding a fruit you can boost the vitamins & minerals in the meal even more!

Eggs are a complete protein, meaning they contain all the essential amino acids, which are the basic components, or "building blocks", of protein. They are called "essential" amino acids because our body cannot make them, so we must get them from the foods we eat.

The great thing about eggs is they provide important nutrients (protein, iron, minerals and B vitamins) in a small volume. This is a bonus for younger children because they have small stomachs and can get full quickly.

If weekday mornings are too pressed for time, you can make eggs on the weekend instead.

A word of caution..... it's best to limit egg yolks to no more than 3 - 4 per week because they are high in saturated fat and cholesterol, two types of fats that are bad for the heart.

EGGS
The 2nd Most
Popular Breakfast
Registered Dietitians
Feed Their Kids

WAFFLES . . .
The 3rd most common breakfast Nutrition Experts feed their kids

Frozen waffles are available in many varieties, some healthy, some not. The unhealthy varieties can have as much as 11 grams of fat and 17 grams of sugar for a 2-waffle serving. Read the Nutrition Facts label carefully and look for options that are low in fat and made with whole wheat flour.

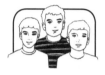 My boys love Eggo NutriGrain Low Fat waffles! They are an easy, tasty way to get a serving of whole grains in the morning, instead of the usual refined white flour in most waffles.

To keep a check on the sugar, limit syrup to 1 tablespoon per waffle. If you buy commercial syrup (vs. 100% Pure Maple Syrup) consider trying the "Light" version. It has half the sugar of regular syrup and most kids don't notice a difference in the taste. Believe me, it's still plenty sweet.

Another option is to try a waffle sandwich with 1 tablespoon Peanut Butter + 1 tablespoon low-sugar jam. All 3 of my boys choose this over syrup on frozen waffles. It makes a healthy, quick, on-the-go breakfast for days when kids (or parents) are running late.

What to look for on the label for *Healthy* Waffles :

Serving Size : 2 waffles
Total Fat : 5 grams or less
Sugar : 6 grams or less
Dietary Fiber: 3 grams or more

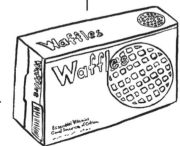

OATMEAL . . .
The 4th most common breakfast Nutrition Experts feed their kids

A quick, microwaveable meal with the benefits of fiber and a serving of whole grains.

The United States Department of Agriculture (USDA) recommends at least 6 servings from the Grain Group for kids 6 to 11 years old and 3 to 5 servings for preschoolers. Of the total servings, at least half should be from whole grains (such as oats, whole wheat bread, brown rice, whole wheat pasta, quinoa, rye or barley). By starting your child's day with a bowl of oatmeal, he'll be off to a good start toward getting all his servings of whole grains for the day.

An added bonus is that oatmeal contains soluble fiber, which can help lower high cholesterol or help maintain healthy cholesterol levels.

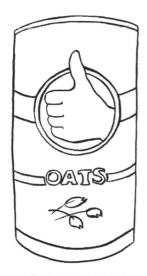

NUTRITION TIP :
To lower the sugar content, microwave whole oats, instead of serving instant, flavored oatmeal packets. That way you can control how much sugar your child gets. By adding 1 teaspoon of brown sugar to plain oats, you cut out 2 to 2 ½ packets (teaspoons) of sugar compared to the sweetened oatmeal! *For variety, crunch, flavor and a nutritional boost, you can add dried fruit and/or nuts* (see recipe page 32).*

OATMEAL
The 4th Most Popular Breakfast
Registered Dietitians Feed Their Kids

Best Oatmeal Ever

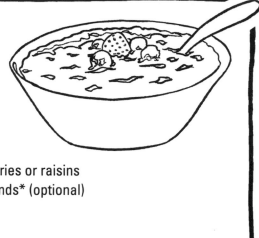

1/3 cup dry oats
2/3 cup water
Sprinkle of cinnamon
1 teaspoon brown sugar
1 tablespoon dried cranberries or raisins
1 tablespoon slivered almonds* (optional)

Nuts are not recommended for children under 4 years old due to a risk of choking.

Preparation :
1. Combine oats, water and cinnamon in a microwaveable bowl.
2. Microwave on HIGH about 2 minutes (time varies per microwave).
3. Add brown sugar, dried fruit and almonds as desired.
4. Stir well, add a splash of nonfat milk and serve.
Makes 1 serving.

Nutrition Information per 2/3-cup serving (with almonds) :
194 calories, 6.6g Total Fat, 1g Saturated Fat, 0mg Cholesterol, 9mg Sodium, 30g Carbohydrate, 4g Fiber, 5g Protein.

Nutrition Information per 2/3-cup serving (no almonds) :
142 calories, 2.0g Total Fat, < 1g Saturated Fat, 0mg Cholesterol, 6mg Sodium, 29g Carbohydrate, 3g Fiber, 3g Protein.

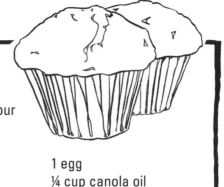

Pumpkin Oat Muffins

Ingredients :

1 ½ cups unbleached all-purpose flour
1 cup quick-cooking oats
1 tablespoon baking powder
½ teaspoon salt
1 teaspoon ground cinnamon
½ teaspoon allspice
¼ teaspoon ground cloves (optional)
¾ cup nonfat milk

1 egg
¼ cup canola oil
¾ cup brown sugar
1 cup canned pumpkin
   (unsweetened)

1/2 cup chopped walnuts* (optional)

Nuts are not recommended for children under 4 years old due to a risk of choking.

Preparation :

1. Heat oven to 400°F. Brush oil in bottom of muffin cups to lightly coat.
2. In a medium bowl combine flour, oats, baking powder, salt and spices. Mix well.
3. In a large bowl, combine milk, egg, oil, brown sugar and pumpkin until well blended.
4. Add flour mixture to egg mixture and stir just until moistened.
5. Fold in nuts.
6. Spoon batter into muffin cups, filling about 2/3 full.
7. Bake at 400°F for 22-25 minutes, or until toothpick inserted comes out clean.
8. Cool 5 minutes, then remove from pan.

Makes 12 muffins.

Nutrition Information per muffin :
205 Calories, 9g Total Fat, 1g Saturated Fat, 18 mg Cholesterol, 190mg Sodium, 28g Carbohydrate, 2g Fiber, 5g Protein.

If your child doesn't like oatmeal, oat muffins are another quick and healthy breakfast option. They're a great on-the-go choice, especially when combined with a fruit and/or yogurt. This recipe is low in sugar and high in nutrition. You can make a double batch and freeze the leftovers for those mornings when you or your kids are running late.

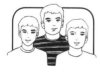

My kids also love these muffins as an after-school snack! They make a great mid-morning snack at school, or even a dessert in a packed lunch or after dinner.

Strategies to increase the Breakfast odds

Is it a challenge to get your kids to eat breakfast? Try these strategies as a start :

1. IT'S THE RULE : When parents set the standard that they *expect* their child to eat breakfast, kids are more likely to make breakfast a habit, rather than an exception.

2. ESTABLISH A WAKE UP TIME : Allow 10 extra minutes to grab a quick breakfast. Sometimes that means getting to bed earlier or setting an alarm or two.

3. PLAN AHEAD : Stock up on easy-to-fix breakfast items, such as frozen waffles, bagels, English muffins, cereals, easy-to-eat fruits (bananas, apples, grapes) and yogurt. If your children are old enough, involve them in the selection, shopping and preparation. Ask them to choose the night before what to have for breakfast.

4. ON-THE-GO OPTIONS : For those kids who won't get out of bed until the absolute last minute, some options that can be eaten on the way to school include :

- · mix of dry cereal & nuts in a baggie + banana
- · waffle sandwich with peanut butter & jelly
- · nonfat yogurt + grapes
- · string cheese + box of raisins (or any dried fruit)
- · bagel with light cream cheese (or peanut butter & jelly)
    made the night before
- · pumpkin oat muffin + fruit

The Bottom Line :

The top 4 breakfasts Nutrition Experts feed their kids are cereal, eggs, waffles and oatmeal. Breakfast is an essential, "must-have" meal because it helps your child fuel up for the day and concentrate better at school! Insist that your child, including tweens and teens, eats breakfast every day. There are many quick, tasty *and* nutritious choices you can provide to help your child start the day off right.

Your Game Plan :

Three examples to get you thinking…

1. I will buy whole grain frozen waffles.
2. I will have my kids choose their breakfast the night before.
3. I will add a fruit to my child's breakfast each morning.

Based on what you've learned in this chapter, what will you change to make breakfast healthier for your child?

New Breakfast Options :

1. _____

2. _____

3. _____

Share Your Thoughts . . .

Please share your experiences with trying new, healthy breakfast foods. Was it easy to make changes? Did you have any difficulties? Are there any great tips or ideas you'd like to share?

**Please go to my website: www.400moms.com
or send me an e-mail at Jill@400moms.com
to share your thoughts and comments!**

CHAPTER 3

SNACKS

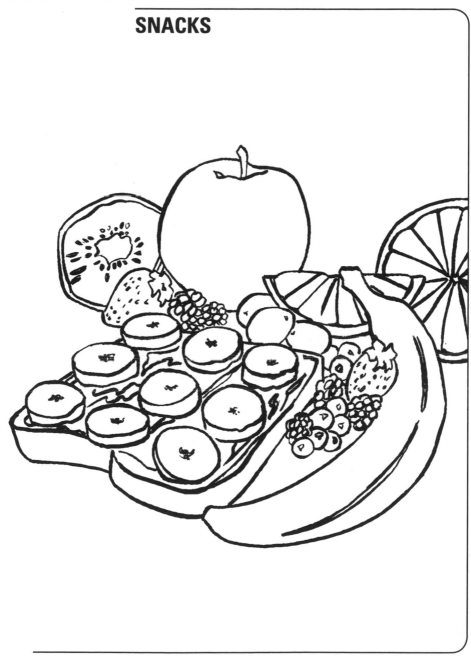

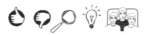

SNACKS . . . Do Kids Need Them?

I'm frequently asked the question, "Do my kids really need snacks?" And I answer wholeheartedly, "YES, but not too much . . ."

Snack time is a great opportunity to round out your child's diet, as well as calm hunger pangs between meals. Children have small stomachs, so they can fill up quickly. The volume they eat at meals usually isn't enough to meet their daily nutrient needs or keep them full enough to make it to the next meal. That's why the right snacks play a very important role in your child's diet.

Snack time is a great time to give your child what she's missing at meals. For example, if your child has cereal and milk for breakfast, offering a fruit mid-morning helps fill in a food group your child missed. If your child doesn't bring or buy milk at school, then serving milk or yogurt as part of his afternoon snack will make up the missing dairy group at lunch.

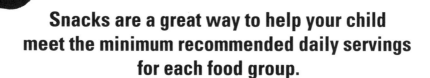

Snacks are a great way to help your child meet the minimum recommended daily servings for each food group.

DID YOU KNOW ...
Beverage, Candy and Fast Food Advertising Expenditures are
Greater than $11 Billion per year?

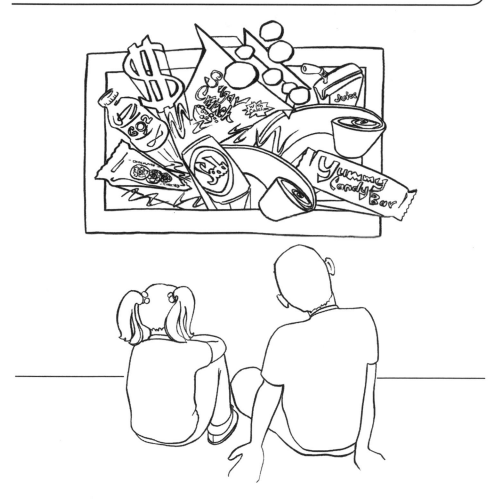

These expenses don't even include dollars spent on product placements in television shows or movies, internet advertising and special promotions. So in reality, the dollars spent are FAR GREATER than $11 billion per year!

DID YOU ALSO KNOW ...
Researchers at Yale University found children consumed *45% more food* when exposed to food advertising?

In another study, researchers at The University of North Carolina, who studied data on more than 31,300 children between the ages of 2 and 18, found that kids are getting 27% of their daily calories from snacks. Unfortunately, the majority of the snack choices are salty snacks, candy, desserts and sweetened beverages, or "empty calories", providing little nutritional value for the calorie cost.

What I take from these studies is that food advertising is contributing to obesity in our children by increasing snack consumption. According to the Centers for Disease Control and Prevention, the prevalence of obesity has more than doubled among children and tripled among teenagers since 1980!

How do you sort through all the hype to find snacks that you know are healthy and that you can feel good about serving to your kids? Well, here are the snacks Nutrition Experts feed their kids.

Top 5 Snacks

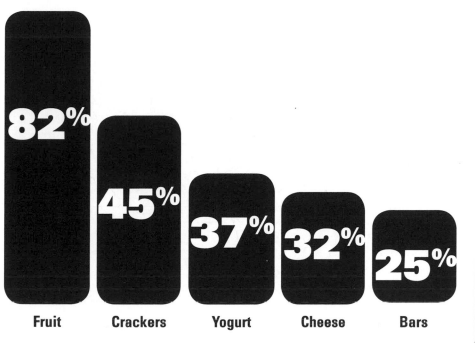

The Top 5 Snacks Registered Dietitians feed their kids are . . .

1. **Fruit**
2. **Crackers**
3. **Yogurt**
4. **Cheese**
5. **Snack Bars** (granola and cereal bars)

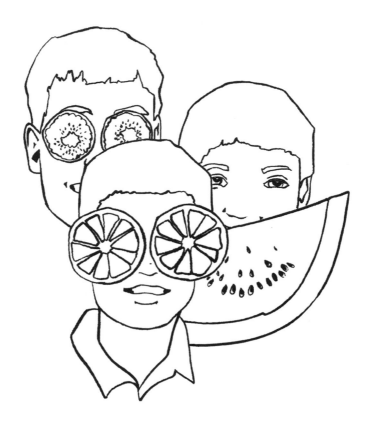

The # 1 snack Registered Dietitians feed their kids is . . . Fruit

82% of Nutrition Experts list fruit (fresh, canned or dried) in the top 4 snacks they serve to their children with apples, bananas and grapes being the most commonly cited fruits.

Why fruit?

It's quick, sweet (which kids love) and full of nutrients, such as fiber, vitamin A, vitamin C, potassium and phytochemicals. Another bonus is that by serving fruit as a snack you can help your child reach the recommended 2 to 4 cups of fruits & vegetables each day.

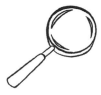

What to look for when choosing fruit :

Fresh, dried or canned fruits are all excellent choices. When serving canned fruit, buy those packed in water or juice and drain the liquid. That way your child is getting the benefit of the whole fruit without the extra sugar from the juice.

Below is a list of fruits that "pack a big punch". They are nutritional powerhouses because they contain antioxidants or nutrients that help prevent and repair damage done to cells and may also improve immunity, *so your child gets sick less often*.

TOP 10 ANTIOXIDANT–RICH FRUITS

Raisins
Blueberries
Blackberries
Strawberries
Raspberries
Plums
Prunes
Oranges
Red Grapes
Cherries

The good news is Nutrition Experts are practical, realistic parents too. They recognize kids like variety and are exposed to the many snack food options available at school and in the supermarket. So what else do they serve regularly?

The # 2 snack Registered Dietitians feed their kids is . . . Crackers

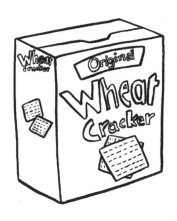
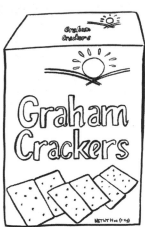
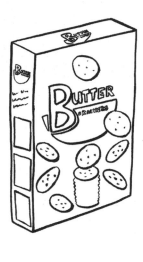

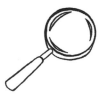

What to look for when choosing crackers :

When parents ask, **"What crackers are healthy?"** I tell them to use the "3 and 3" Rule. The healthiest options have at least **3 grams of Fiber** and no more than **3 grams of Total Fat** (per one-ounce serving).

Some parents say it's challenging to find crackers their child will eat that are *both low in fat and high in fiber*. So on *page 48* I created a list of my "Best Picks" that meet the criteria for low in fat, high in fiber, or both. That way you can decide what your nutrition priority is: low in fat, high in fiber, or BOTH.

Buyers Beware . . .

Tip # 1 : Check the label carefully

In reading the Nutrition Facts label, pay close attention to the **serving size** information. The standard serving size for crackers is 1 ounce, which can also be shown as 28-32 grams. This is where it can get tricky. Some companies list a serving size as 14-16 grams, which is only ½ ounce. Why do they do this? To make the nutrition numbers look better.

For example, Nabisco Ritz Crackers lists a serving as 5 crackers (16g). This makes the calories, total fat and all the other nutrients *appear* lower because this is only half of a serving. Tricky, I know.

So instead of the Total Fat being 4.5 grams as listed on the label, it's really double that, or 9 grams of Total Fat and 160 calories for a standard 30 grams (or 1-oz. serving size). The same applies to the Reduced Fat Ritz crackers, which are really 5 grams of Total Fat and *not* a low fat cracker.

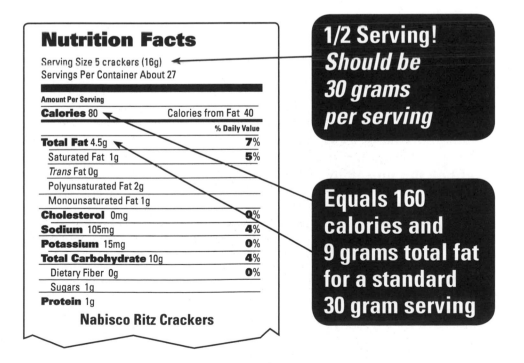

Tip # 2 : Don't get fooled by "whole grain" claims

Since the USDA guidelines recommend half of our daily servings of grains come from whole grains, choosing crackers made with whole grains is a great way to help your child get those servings. Just make sure what you *think* is a whole grain cracker really *is* a whole grain cracker. Some companies are using whole grain claims on the front of the package as a marketing strategy. Oftentimes the amount of whole grain in these crackers is so small it's insignificant.

For example, on the front of the box of Ritz Whole Wheat crackers it says "with 5g Whole Grain per serving". Sounds like a lot, doesn't it? Most consumers think 5 grams of whole grain is the same as 5 grams of fiber. It's not. What the box doesn't tell you is that in order for the crackers to count as a whole grain serving, you need **16 grams of whole grain**. By taking a closer look at this label, you'll see that a serving of crackers has < 1 gram of fiber and the first ingredient is unbleached enriched flour, which is a fancy name for white flour.

Another example is Multigrain Club Crackers. They must be healthier than the original, right? After all, they're "multigrain". Wrong! By taking a closer look at this label it reveals that a serving provides less than 1 gram of fiber and the first ingredient is enriched flour, same as the Ritz Crackers.

An example of a cracker that *does* contain whole grains is Triscuits. The package claim says "Baked Whole Grain Wheat Crackers". A closer look at the label reveals that a serving of Reduced Fat Triscuits provides 2.5grams of fiber and the first ingredient is whole grain soft white winter wheat.

So how do you know if crackers really count as a whole grain? 1st: check the ingredient list. 2nd: check the fiber

The first ingredient should have the keyword "whole". There are many grains that could be listed, but a few examples are whole wheat flour, whole grain rye, whole oat flour, whole grain barley, or oats. Fiber is a little trickier because some manufacturers are now adding fiber that may not come from a whole grain. However, it's still a useful checkpoint, after the ingredient list. As a reminder, ingredients that are NOT a whole grain include enriched wheat flour, wheat flour or enriched flour.

Tip # 3 : Watch out for sodium

Snack foods are known for being high in sodium–and crackers are no exception. On average, they have about 250mg of sodium per 1-ounce serving, but range from 50mg to 340mg per serving. To help give you some perspective, I've listed several foods and the amount of sodium in these products:

	Serving	Sodium Content
Chips	1 oz.	110-300mg
Pretzels	1 oz.	250-560mg
Microwave Popcorn	2 cups	90-200mg
Sliced bread	1 slice	150-170mg
Cereal	1 cup	0-360mg

The practical side of me knows and understands how difficult it can be to meet all the healthy criteria for snacks. Adding yet another nutrient to check on the label may be too much, and if so, I suggest you focus on low fat and high fiber choices first.

SUMMARY

When choosing crackers, low in fat and high in fiber is ideal. Low fat crackers with 2 grams of fiber is a **big improvement** over white bread, chips, typical crackers and other snack foods on the shelf. To make your shopping easier, I've listed my "Best Picks" on the next page.

Jill's Best Picks :
Best Crackers

Manufacturer	BRAND	Grams of FIBER	Grams of FAT	Sodium (mg)
RyKrisp	Seasoned	6	3	180
Ak-mak	Original	4	2	223
Kashi	Heart To Heart	4	3.5	85
Nabisco	Triscuits Reduced Fat Plain	3	2.5	160
Trader Joes	Reduced Guilt Wheat Wafers	3	2.5	210
Kellogg's	Special K - Savory Herb	3	3	210
Kellogg's	Special K - Multi-Grain	3	3	220
Trader Joes	Multi-Grain Pita Bites	3	3.5	170
Nabisco	Triscuits Hint Of Salt	3	4	50
Nabisco	Triscuits Reduced Fat Flavored	3	4	140
Kashi	TLC 7-Grain	3	3.5	160
Nabisco	Wheat Thins - Reduced Fat	3	3.5	230
Trader Joes	Multi-Grain & Flaxseed	2	2	170
Trader Joes	Reduced Guilt Wheat Crisps	2	4	150

The "Best Picks" crackers are listed with the *healthiest choice at the top*. I ranked the crackers based on the amount of Fiber first and Total Fat second because it's really important to increase the number of whole grains our kids are eating. There are a few crackers that have enough fiber to make this list, but are too high in fat. I limited the "Best Picks" to those that had no more than 4 grams of Total Fat per serving to ensure all choices on this list were healthy for both total fat and fiber.

As I mentioned earlier, the ideal nutrition combination for crackers is "3 and 3", or at least **3 grams of Fiber** and no more than **3 grams of Total Fat per serving.** However, being a practical Mom, I included some choices that are close to the ideal because I believe they're still a healthy choice.

NOTE: if multiple flavors are available, an average of all varieties was calculated for fiber, fat and sodium. If you find brands that don't make either list, it could be that they're not available throughout the country or they fall into a "grey zone": high in fiber, but too high in fat or low in fiber and medium in fat. Use the "3 and 3" rule to see if they make the "Best Picks" list.

Jill's Worst Picks :
Worst Cracker Choices

Manufacturer	BRAND	Grams of FAT	Grams of FIBER	Sodium (mg)
Keebler	Townhouse Original	10	1	260
Nabisco	Ritz	9	< 1	260
Nabisco	Better Cheddars	8	< 1	290
Nabisco	Chicken in a Buscuit	8	< 1	240
Sunshine	Cheezits	8	< 1	230
Nabisco	Sociables	7	0	240
Nabisco	Vegatable Thins	7	1	320
Dare	Breton	7	1	265
Pepperidge Farm	Harvest Wheat	7	1	250
Nabisco	Wheatsworth	7	2	360
Carr's	Whole Wheat	7	2	175
Nabisco	Cheese Nips	6	< 1	340
Keebler	Original Club	6	< 1	250
Keebler	Multigrain Club	6	< 1	240
Nabisco	Ritz Pretzel Rounds	6	1	340
Pepperidge Farm	Cheese Crisps	6	2	270
Milton's	Multigrain	5	< 1	200
Carr's	Rosemary	5	< 1	280
Peperidg Farm	Goldfish	5	1	250
Pepperidge Farm	Goldfish - Whole Grain	5	2	250
Pepperidge Farm	Wheat Crisps	5	2	240
Nabisco	Wheat Thins - Original	5	3	230
Nabisco	Wheat Thins - Multigrain	4.5	3	200
Sunshine	Cheezits - Reduced Fat	4.5	< 1	250
Sunshine	Cheezit Snack Mix	4.5	1	310

The "Worst Picks" crackers are ranked with the *unhealthiest choice at the top*. For this list, I used Total Fat as the #1 criteria and Fiber as the #2 criteria because :

1. The fiber is so dismally low in most of the choices.

2. The fat is so high for many of the choices that even if the crackers were a good source of fiber, I wouldn't recommend them.

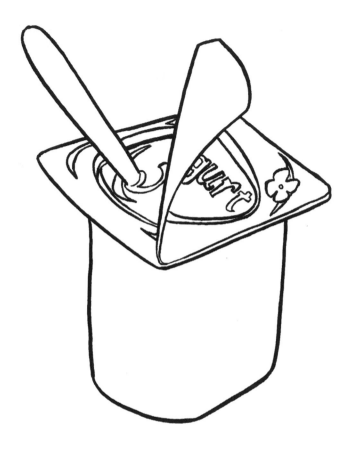

The # 3 snack Registered Dietitians feed their kids is . . . Yogurt

Why do Nutrition Experts give their kids yogurt? First of all, it's sweet, so most kids are happy about that and don't need a lot of convincing to eat it!

Second, it provides calcium, vitamin D and some protein, making it a more nutritious choice than many other snack foods. Another bonus is that by offering yogurt, you help your child get a serving from the Dairy Group, whereas chips, cookies and most granola bars don't meet any food group servings.

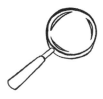

What to look for when choosing yogurt :
Just like most snacks, there are MANY yogurt choices on the shelf, and some are healthier than others. Choose brands with 20% calcium or more.

Sugar

Yogurt contains lactose, which is a naturally-occurring sugar in milk. The amount of naturally-occurring sugar in a 6 oz. container of plain yogurt is about 10 grams. However, most flavored yogurts contain added sugars. When reading the Nutrition Facts label, any amount of sugar above 10 grams will be added sugar. The goal is to buy yogurts that are as close to 10 grams of sugar as possible to avoid unnecessary extra sugar. The natural sugar content in 4oz yogurt cups is about 6.5 grams per container.

Calcium

One great health benefit of yogurt is that it can be an excellent source of calcium if you choose carefully. When reading the Nutrition Facts label, choose yogurts with *at least* 20% calcium per 6 oz. container - or 15% per 4oz container. Some brands and flavors contain 30% calcium, which is even better.

On *page 54* I've ranked the yogurt brands based on calcium and vitamin D first, and no more than the equivalent of 20 grams of sugar for a 6 oz. container, which is double the sugar of plain yogurt. Many varieties that are pourable or that come in small tubes are quite high in sugar, so choices such as Yoplait Gogurt, Yokids Squeezers, Danimals Smoothie, Danimals tube didn't make the list because if they were in a 6 oz. container they would have as much as 25-30 grams of sugar, which is 4-5 packets of added sugar!

Keep in mind that some varieties are sweetened with artificial sweetener, and some parents are opposed to providing foods with artificial sweeteners to their children. If that's a concern for you, check the Nutrition Facts labels and choose yogurts that have *at least* **20% calcium and 20% Vitamin D** as the priority over sugar.

Jill's Best Picks :
Best Yogurt Choices

BRAND	Size	% Calcium	% Vit-D	Grams of Sugar
Yoplait - Greek	6 oz.	35	20	20
Weight Watchers*	6 oz.	30	30	11
Stonyfield - Organic	6 oz.	30	20	17
Yoplait - Thick & Creamy	6 oz.	30	20	28
Yobaby	4 oz.	25	25	13
Cascade Fresh	6 oz.	25	0	16
Trader Joe's - Organic Greek Style	6 oz.	25	0	17
Yoplait - Light*	6 oz.	20	20	10
Yoplait - Simplait*	6 oz.	20	0	24
Yoplait Kids	3 oz.	20	20	9
Dannon - Light & Fit*	6 oz.	15	15	11
Stonyfield Yokids	4 oz.	15	25	13
Yoplait Whips	6 oz.	15	10	21
Dannon Oikos	5.3 oz.	15	15	18
Dannon Activa	4oz.	15	10	17
Chobani - Greek Yogurt	6 oz.	15	0	20
Yoplait - Greek 100 Calories	5.3 oz.	10	20	9
Trader Joe's Greek Style Nonfat	5.3 oz.	0	0	14

* sweetened with artificial sweeteners, such as aspartame, sucralose or acesulfame potassium. For some brands the sugar content varies from flavor to flavor, so the number listed is an average of several flavors.

Since there are other ways to get calcium besides yogurt and milk, I want to take a few minutes to talk about how much calcium your child needs and how to determine if he or she is getting enough. The amount of calcium recommended depends on age and increases as your child gets older.

CALCIUM NEEDS

Age 1 to 3 years old = 700mg/day
Age 4 to 8 years old = 1000mg/day
Age 9 to 18 years old = 1300mg/day

The amount of calcium on the Nutrition Facts label will be listed as a percentage, instead of milligrams(mg), as shown in the table.

The percentage is based on a reference amount of 1,000mg of calcium. For example, the label below shows this product has 20% calcium. If you then multiply 20% X 1,000mg, you'll know that this product has 200mg of calcium.

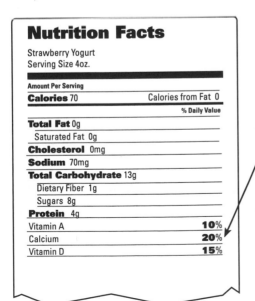

Nutrition Facts

Strawberry Yogurt
Serving Size 4oz.

Amount Per Serving	
Calories 70	Calories from Fat 0
	% Daily Value
Total Fat 0g	
Saturated Fat 0g	
Cholesterol 0mg	
Sodium 70mg	
Total Carbohydrate 13g	
Dietary Fiber 1g	
Sugars 8g	
Protein 4g	
Vitamin A	**10**%
Calcium	**20**%
Vitamin D	**15**%

When your child eats a yogurt with 20% calcium, he gets 200mg of the total calcium he needs for the day.

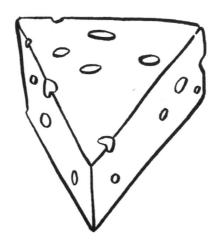

The # 4 snack Registered Dietitians feed their kids is . . . Cheese

Although cheese sometimes gets a bad rap because it's high in fat, for growing, healthy kids cheese is a great snack in moderation. If you buy cheeses that are made from 2% milk or part-skim milk you decrease how much unhealthy saturated fat your child gets, but keep the healthy protein and calcium the same.

When thinking about the five food groups, cheese is part of the Dairy Group, but also has valuable protein. By combining cheese with another food group, such as fruit or whole grain crackers, you help your child get 2 different food groups in one snack.

A quick snack my kids love is Mini Pizzas

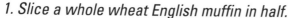

1. Slice a whole wheat English muffin in half.
2. Spread 1 tablespoon spaghetti sauce on each half.
3. Sprinkle shredded part-skim mozzarella cheese on top.

Pop in the toaster oven and toast for a warm, crunchy, filling snack!

The # 5 snack Registered Dietitians feed their kids is . . . Snack Bars

A very popular choice among kids, but challenging as a parent if "healthy" is what you're looking for! There has been an explosion of brands and varieties, most of which are high in fat, sugar, or both. As a matter of fact, some snack bars have as much as 13 grams of fat or 15 grams of sugar. These bars definitely don't qualify as a healthy snack. However, as an alternative to other desserts, such as candy and cookies, some snack bars can be lower in fat and sugar, and higher in fiber when chosen carefully. *In my quest to find a healthy snack bar, here's what I found . . .*

Jill's Best Picks :
Best Snack Bars

BRAND	Grams of FIBER	Grams of SUGAR	Grams of FAT
Kellogg's Fibre Plus Antioxidants	9	7	4-5
Kashi TLC Chewy Bars	4	5-8	2-5
Kashi Crunchy Bars (2-Bars)	4	8-10	6
Kellogg's Special K Bars	3	6-8	1.5-2

(If the brand has multiple flavors, then a range is listed to include all flavors.)

DID YOU KNOW . . .

The most popular granola bars are only slightly better than Kellogg's Pop Tarts? Nobody would say a Pop Tart is a healthy choice, but many parents believe snack bars are healthy. The truth is most snack bars are just like cookies: low in fiber and high in sugar, unless you're choosing the "Best Picks" snack bars above.

Jill's Worst Picks :
Worst Snack Bars

BRAND	Grams of FIBER	Grams of SUGAR	Grams of FAT
Nature Valley Chewy Yogurt Bars	1	14	4
Nature Valley Trail Mix	1 - 2	13 - 15	4
Nature Valley Sweet & Salty Nut	1 - 2	11 - 13	7 - 9
Quaker Chewy Dips Granola Bar	1 - 2	12 - 13	5 - 6
Nutrigrain Cereal Bars	3	11 - 12	3
Nature Valley Roasted Nut Crunch	2	6	13

These bars make the Worst List because they're high in sugar, high in fat, low in fiber, or all 3.

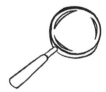

What to look for when choosing snack bars :

Check the Nutrition Facts label and choose varieties with :

2 grams fiber (or more)

5 grams total fat (or less)

8 grams of sugar (or less)

What's In Your Cupboard?

Go to your kitchen and open the cupboards. What do you see? What kinds of snacks currently fill your shelves? Count the number of healthy snacks your child has to choose from. Many parents know they have an abundance of unhealthy snacks available, but have trouble coming up with healthy snack ideas they think their kids will eat. One strategy I recommend is to combine two food groups when making a snack. For example, cereal + milk provides a serving from the Grains Group + a serving from the Dairy Group. Another example is fruit + string cheese, which provides a serving from the Fruit Group and a serving from the Dairy Group, helping to "round out" your child's diet and increase the chances of getting all the recommended daily servings.

I've created a list of healthy snacks Nutrition Experts feed their kids (on the next page). You can use this list to stock your cupboard and refrigerator or refer to it when you go grocery shopping.

A Word About PEANUT BUTTER . . .

Many Registered Dietitians offer peanut butter with crackers, fruit or celery as a snack option. Peanut butter is nutritious, adds variety, and can help encourage a child to choose a healthy food more often because it tastes better with peanut butter on it.

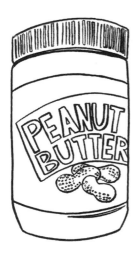

Many parents think peanut butter is mostly protein, but it's actually mostly fat (77% of the calories come from fat, while only 17% of the calories come from protein). The type of fats in peanut butter are mostly monounsaturated and polyunsaturated fats, which are "heart-healthy" fats. Almond butter and cashew butter are also healthy choices.

Children need some fat in their diet for healthy growth and development, so peanut butter is an excellent choice. Peanut butter is a "calorie-dense" food, or a lot of calories for a small volume. Unless your child is extremely active and needs extra calories, it's important to keep the serving size to 1 - 2 tablespoons because too much fat can contribute to too much weight gain.

25 HEALTHY SNACK IDEAS

Graham Crackers + Milk

Light Microwave Popcorn

Fresh Fruit

Vegetables & Dip

Pita Bread with Hummus

Rice Cakes with Peanut Butter

Dried Fruit

Low Fat Crackers with Peanut Butter

Deli Meat Rolls

Yogurt + Raisins

Cereal + Milk

Nuts (if your child is over 4 years old)

Pumpkin Oat Muffins (see recipe on *page 33*)

Magic Muffins (see recipe on *page 60*)

Trail Mix (see recipe on next page)

Applesauce or Fruit Cup

Fruit Smoothie (see recipe *page 164*)

Beef Jerky or Turkey Jerky

Leftover Pasta with Sauce

Whole Wheat Toast with Peanut Butter

English Muffin Pizza (see recipe on *page 54*)

Cottage Cheese with Fruit

Crackers with Tuna

Pretzels

Oatmeal

½ Bagel with Cream Cheese

Go to www.400moms.com to print a copy to put on your refrigerator.

EASY SNACK RECIPES . . .

For those who like to have homemade, easy-to-grab snacks on hand, here are a couple of my kids' favorite choices.

TRAIL MIX for KIDS

Ingredients :
½ cup dried cranberries
½ cup raisins
½ cup almonds or peanuts*
1 ½ cups low sugar cereal
(i.e. Kix, Chex, Crispix, Life, Cheerios, Oat Squares)

* For children under 4 years old, omit nuts to prevent choking.

Preparation :

1. Combine all ingredients in a medium sized bowl. Mix thoroughly.

2. Pour into a medium-sized, air-tight container or scoop ½ cup servings into re-sealable baggies or small plastic containers.
Makes 6 servings.

Nutrition Information per 1/2 -cup serving :
165 calories, 6g Total Fat, <1g Saturated Fat, 0mg Cholesterol, 26g Carbohydrate, 3g Fiber, 3g Protein, 73mg Sodium.

This snack is just what mom wants and kids need: a good source of fiber, filling and sweet! You can add it to a lunch bag as a snack or dessert or serve after school with milk or fruit.

I do have a confession to make… my 3 boys like this recipe even better when it includes M&M's. However, they will gladly eat it without them! Every once in a while, I will surprise them by adding ¼ cup M&M's or chocolate chips as a treat. It adds less than a Tablespoon to each serving, but they love the bite of chocolate.

MAGIC MUFFINS

Ingredients :

1 egg
½ cup packed brown sugar
¼ cup canola oil
¼ cup nonfat milk
1 teaspoon vanilla
1 ¼ cups unbleached all-purpose flour
2 teaspoons baking powder
1 teaspoon ground cinnamon
½ teaspoon ground allspice
½ cup packed shredded carrots (1 medium to large carrot)
½ cup packed shredded apple (about ½ apple)
1/3 cup dried cranberries
1/3 cupchopped walnuts

Preparation :

1. Heat oven to 375°F. Brush oil in muffin cups to lightly coat.
2. In a large mixing bowl, combine egg, brown sugar, oil, milk and vanilla until well blended.
3. In a separate bowl, combine flour, baking powder, cinnamon and allspice. Add to egg mixture and stir just until dry ingredients are moistened.
4. Stir in carrots, apple, cranberries and nuts.
5. Spoon batter into muffin cups, filling about ½ full.
6. Bake at 375°F for 15-17 minutes, or until toothpick inserted comes out clean. Cool 5 minutes, then remove from pan.

Makes 12 muffins.

Nutrition Information per muffin :
169 calories, 7g Total Fat,< 1g Saturated Fat, 18 mg Cholesterol, 76mg Sodium, 24g Carbohydrate, 1g Fiber, 3g Protein

Note: To make these muffins even healthier, use 3/4 cup white flour and 1/2 cup whole wheat flour.

These muffins serve as a great example of what a serving or portion of muffin *should be*, compared to what your kids see in the bakery or grocery store. To learn more about portion sizes, go to Chapter 11.

The Bottom Line :

The top 4 snacks Nutrition Experts feed their kids are fruit, crackers, yogurt and cheese. Snacks are an *essential* part of your child's diet. What type of snacks you offer matters a lot. It determines whether your child gets mostly fat and sugar from snacks or gets important nutrients that are otherwise missed and not made up at later meals.

Your Game Plan :

Three examples to get you thinking…

1. I will serve fruit at afternoon snack each day.
2. I will buy "Best Picks" for crackers and snack bars.
3. I will have my child choose from the Healthy Snack Ideas (*page 60*).

Based on what you've learned in this chapter, what will you change to make snacks healthier for your child?

New Snack Ideas :

1. _____

2. _____

3. _____

Share Your Thoughts . . .

I would love to hear what new, healthy snacks you've added to your cupboards and refrigerator! What are your kids' favorite healthy snacks? Have you or your kids created any of your own snack recipes? Have you noticed any benefits from making the changes? Was it easy to do or did you have some difficulties? Are there any great tips or ideas you'd like to share?

Please go to my website: www.400moms.com or send me an e-mail at Jill@400moms.com to share your thoughts and comments!

CHAPTER 4

LUNCH

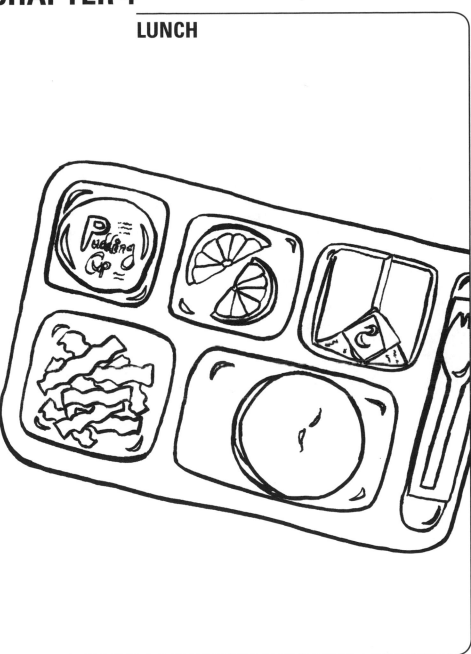

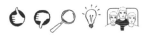

LUNCH . . .
To Buy Or Not To Buy?

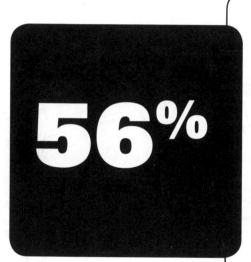

56%

When I surveyed over 400 Nutrition Experts about the lunches they provide their children, 56% of Registered Dietitians said they buy School Lunches for their children 1 day per week OR NEVER!

Well, that's a strong statement!

Over half of the responders significantly limit how often their children eat the lunch provided at school. At first I was surprised, but then again, I don't buy the school lunch for my kids either.

Why?

Because most school lunches are a nutrition bomb— too high in total fat, saturated fat and sodium and too low in vitamins and fiber. Although there are more school districts in the country developing school lunch programs with high nutrition standards, the great majority of schools continue providing the usual choices: chicken nuggets, cheeseburger sliders, nachos, pizza, chicken filet sandwich (breaded & fried, of course), hot dogs and corn dogs. Unfortunately, the National School Lunch Program is providing these unhealthy meals to more than *32 million* students nationwide.

To make matters worse, a recent study found that between 2006 and 2010 almost **half** of public and private schools surveyed sold sweet or salty snack foods during the school day. This clearly indicates that many schools are not listening to messages from health advocates urging schools to limit the types of food available outside of mealtimes. Schools most likely to sell chips, candy, cookies and other unhealthy snack foods were located in the South where obesity rates are the highest. So not only does your child receive a high fat lunch, but he can pack in more high fat, high sugar items by purchasing snacks that the school justifies by calling it "fundraising".

However, there's some good news: healthy changes are on the horizon! In December 2010, Congress passed The Healthy Hunger-Free Kids Act, which includes legislation to update the nutrition standards for breakfast and lunch meals to provide healthier, more nutritious food options at school. The legislation also includes provisions to educate children about making healthy food choices and teach them about healthy habits for a lifetime. Some of the standards are already being implemented throughout the country, but it will take years before we see the benefits of this legislation. Schools have an important role in helping our children be healthy, but so do parents!

As a parent, you need to do your part to provide healthy, low fat lunch options.

By offering healthy choices, together we can begin to decrease the rates of obesity, diabetes and heart disease in our children.

Let's look at a School Lunch compared to a Packed Lunch Bag :

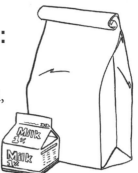

School Lunch - Chicken Nuggets, Tater Tots, Canned Peaches, 1% Milk

Packed Lunch - Turkey Sandwich on Wheat Bread, Fresh Fruit, Nonfat Milk

Why it's Better - Less fat, less sodium, more fiber, more vitamins, less sugar

How the numbers stack up :

This school lunch example has 24 grams extra fat, 4 grams saturated fat and 195 extra unhealthy calories. Picture yourself spreading *4 tablespoons of mayonnaise* on your child's turkey sandwich for lunch. That is the equivalent of 24 grams of extra fat the school lunch provides in the above example.

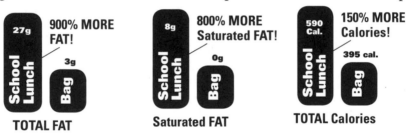

Just in case you're wondering, the cheeseburgers, nachos, corn dogs, pizza, and other school lunches previously mentioned stack up the same unhealthy numbers as the chicken nuggets and tater tots used in this example. Although we know kids need to gain some weight as they grow, if your child is consistently eating 195 extra calories from a lunch meal and doesn't burn off those extra calories, then he or she will gain too much weight.

For example, a child who weighs about 60 pounds would have to run or play an active game like soccer or basketball for *an extra 45 minutes* above and beyond his or her usual activity for the day to burn off the extra 195 calories. It isn't important to know exactly how many calories your child eats at a meal, but it makes it pretty obvious why kids are overweight if they're eating chicken nuggets, cheeseburgers, nachos, pizza and corn dogs on a daily basis.

Although the school lunch is a *very* convenient option, most Nutrition Experts choose to pack a lunch for their child over the convenience of buying a lunch that is nutritionally inadequate at best and harmful to your child's health at worst. **By packing a lunch for your child, you have control of how much sugar, fat and calories go into the bag.**

In the comparison between the school lunch of chicken nuggets and the packed turkey sandwich lunch, the health benefits of the packed lunch are impressive. However, a packed lunch can have the same pitfalls of a school lunch (too much fat, sodium and unhealthy calories) depending on what foods get packed in the bag.

The following table provides healthy substitutions for more traditional lunch choices. A few minor changes can significantly lower the fat and increase the fiber and vitamins in the lunch you pack for your child.

Throw Away . . .	Replace With . . .
Bologna sandwich with mayonnaise on white bread	Ham or turkey sandwich with mustard on wheat bread, or tuna pita sandwich
Chips	Pretzels, reduced fat crackers, light popcorn, veggies & low fat dip
Fruit cup in syrup	Fresh or dried fruit
Cream-filled cookies, Chocolate chip cookies or candy	Low fat pudding, homemade muffins, nonfat yogurt, homemade trail mix, fruit, vanilla wafers, fig bars, animal crackers, graham crackers
Fruit drinks, juice, soda or energy drinks	Water, nonfat milk or 1% milk

Keep in mind that the prepackaged kids' lunch meals available in the deli section of the grocery store don't count as a healthy "packed lunch". They may be convenient, but they pack one big, unhealthy punch! They're high in fat, sugar, sodium and empty calories. These meals typically include processed meat or cheese, low fiber bread or crackers, no fruit and candy for dessert. The sodium ranges from **500mg to 900mg**, and the sugar is as high as **45 grams** because of the candy and juice! These meals make the school lunch seem healthy.…At least the school lunch offers a fruit and milk option instead of candy and a juice bag!

Top 4 Lunch Entrees

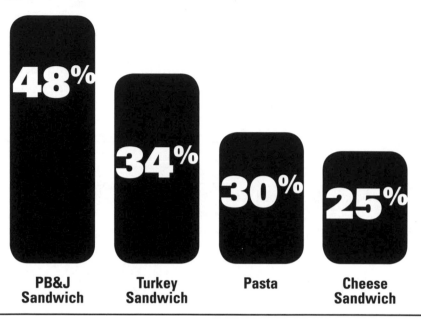

PB&J Sandwich	Turkey Sandwich	Pasta	Cheese Sandwich
48%	34%	30%	25%

The Top-4 Lunch entrees Registered Dietitians prepare for their kids are :

 # 1 : Peanut Butter Sandwich or Peanut Butter & Jelly Sandwich (48%)

 # 2 : Turkey Sandwich (34%)

 # 3 : Pasta (30%)

 # 4 : Grilled Cheese Sandwich, Cheese Sandwich, Quesadilla or Cheese & Crackers (25%)

When packing a lunch from home, I recommend taking time to brainstorm healthy options with your child to find foods and snacks he or she is willing to eat.

By engaging kids in the process, they're more likely to eat what is packed and less likely to complain about what you packed for them.

Before brainstorming it's important to establish that junk foods will not be a daily choice in the lunch, but can be incorporated once in a while. As the parent you need to decide what "once in awhile" will be. I've found that kids are usually willing to eat the healthy choices most of the time if occasionally they get a choice that is less healthy. After all, lunch is as much social as it is nourishing.

Getting complaints about "the same-old, same-old"?

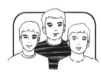

Some kids are perfectly happy having the same lunch every day. When one of my boys was in third grade he had half a peanut butter sandwich, fruit, crackers and water for lunch every school day. My preference would have been that he had more variety, but he was happy and his lunch got eaten, so I didn't complain. He got plenty of variety at breakfast, snacks and dinner each day, as well as weekend lunches.

I can tell you 8 years later he's healthy and thriving. He eats much more variety now, so no harm done, and it was much healthier than the school lunch option!

Other kids, however, complain that lunch is boring if they have a sandwich every day.

So, in addition to the old standby, peanut butter and jelly, these kids might enjoy sandwich variations, such as a pita sandwich filled with tuna or deli ham or a tortilla wrap filled with grilled chicken, shredded lettuce, diced cucumber and pickles. You might try pasta salad or last night's pasta leftovers as a quick and easy lunch option as well. When cleaning up after dinner, store the pasta in individual containers that can go right into the lunch bag (with a cold pack) in the morning.

What's For Lunch?

Many Nutrition Experts listed some less traditional, yet nutritious lunch ideas. These are entrée suggestions, so be sure to include a fruit and/or vegetable along with the entrée.

- Rice Cakes + Peanut Butter or Almond Butter
- Whole grain crackers + cheese slices
- Leftover chicken drumstick + roll
- Apple + reduced-fat cheese stick
- Hard-boiled egg + wheat crackers
- Bean & cheese burrito
- Pita bread sandwich with almond butter & honey
- Leftover chicken & rice mixture
- Chicken Noodle Soup (in a thermos) + whole grain crackers
- Leftover Chili (in an insulated food jar) + whole grain roll
- Leftover pasta salad (see recipe *page 102*)
- Black beans & rice
- Pizza Wrap (see recipe *page 76*)
- Low fat refried beans & salsa + whole grain crackers
- Cottage cheese mixed with peaches or pineapple chunks
- Cup of yogurt mixed with Grapenuts cereal or low fat granola
- Leftover Pasta with parmesan cheese (see recipe *page 78*)
- Peanut butter & apple wrap (see recipe *page 77*)

What Else to Pack in the Lunch Bag?

Depending on age and growth spurts, many kids are hungry for a snack at recess or need the extra food at lunch, along with their entrée and fruit.

Here are some snack ideas mentioned by Nutrition Experts to send with your child to eat at recess or as part of lunch.

· Dried fruit (i.e. apricots, mango, raisins, blueberries or cranberries)
· Fruit salad
· Apple slices with peanut butter
· Unsweetened applesauce or fruit cup in juice
· Whole grain crackers (at least 2-3 grams fiber/serving)
· Nuts: almonds, peanuts, pistachios
· Celery with peanut butter
· Nonfat yogurt (frozen or refrigerated)
· Homemade Trail Mix (see recipe *page 59*)
· Baby carrots, cucumbers, celery, bell pepper slices or snap peas with homemade Ranch dip (see recipe *page 141*)
· Fruit slices dipped in vanilla or lemon yogurt
· Fruit leather (made of 100% dried fruit, no sugar or juice)
· Dry cereal - such as Multi-Grain Cheerios, Kix, Life, Crispix, etc.
· Pretzels & Popcorn

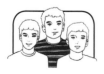

My kids would complain about fruit "getting mushed" or being too warm by lunchtime, so they are big fans of dried fruit and dry cereal as snacks in their lunch. Fruit cups and fruit leathers work well for the same reason, but read labels carefully and avoid brands that contain added sugar, juice or juice concentrate in addition to the natural fruit sugar.

"Should I include a dessert?"
A frequently asked question by many parents!

With the numerous treats that creep into a school day (cupcakes for a classmate's birthday, a candy treat from a teacher or parent helper, cookies after school at a friend's house), the unplanned desserts can become excessive and difficult to monitor or control. Consequently, I suggest skipping dessert at lunch.

Two other options are to include a dessert at lunch 2 or 3 days per week (instead of daily) or to have dessert on the weekend when additional sweets are less likely to sneak in. If your child plays on sports teams, parents frequently provide an after-game snack. Why is it that these snacks are usually a dessert or other junk food? In this case, you can substitute the after-game snack for the dessert you would have served at home.

If you choose to include a dessert in your child's lunch, be careful of the portion size. Some prepackaged cookie packs contain as much as 270 calories per pack! Although convenient, these cookie packs, which make the "Worst Picks" list on the next page, are too large of a portion, full of fat and sugar (empty calories), and crowd out important nutrients.

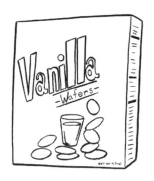

I recommend 100 to 150 calories for a dessert serving.

For example, Nabisco Reduced fat Nilla Wafers are on the "Best Picks" list (see *page 153*) and in checking the Nutrition Facts label it shows a serving size of 8 cookies is 120 calories. This serving fits within the guideline of 100 to 150 calories for a dessert serving and helps you decide how many cookies to pack in your child's lunch. I know for some parents convenience is essential; if so, look for the smaller cookie packs and check the Nutrition Facts label to find options that are within the 100 - 150 calorie range per bag.

Jill's Worst Picks :
Worst Cookie Packs

BRAND	# of Calories	Grams of FAT	Grams of SUGAR
Nabisco Oreos	270	11	23
Nabisco NutterButter Peanut Butter Sandwich	260	11	17
Nabisco Snackwells	210	5	18
Keebler Deluxe mini Rainbow	200	10	14
Famous Amos Chocolate Chip	200	10	13
Keebler Mini Fudge Stripes	200	9	13
Nabisco Fig Newtons	200	4	23
Nabisco Chips Ahoy Choc. Chip	190	9	13

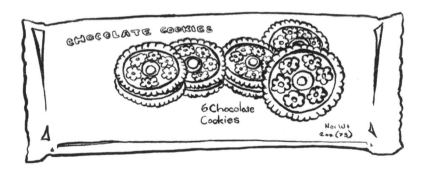

Instead of choosing these large cookie packs, buy the box or package of cookies that make the "Best Picks" list on *page 153* in Chapter 8 and include a serving of cookies in a resealable, reusable baggie. Not only are you helping the environment by decreasing packaging waste, but you're also teaching your kids what an appropriate portion size is for dessert.

"Can I have the best of both worlds?"

In today's busy world most parents are looking for both convenience & healthy choices when providing lunch for a child.

 ## Here are a few ideas to consider....

1. Identify days when the school menu choice.

If your school serves healthy options, plan for those days to be "buy lunch" days and pack a lunch on the other days, or allow your child to make the choice of which day to buy lunch.

2. Choose 1 or 2 days that will be "buy lunch" days.

Even if they're not the healthiest choice, at least the frequency of unhealthy lunches can be limited to 1 or 2 days and healthy lunches can make up the remaining days of the week.

3. Enlist the help of your child.

Make it a routine that your child partially packs his or her lunch the night before, choosing the fruit, vegetable and snack portion, so that in the morning the only items to add are the entrée portion and milk or water. There are two great benefits here: it simplifies lunch making in the morning and it teaches your child how to create a healthy lunch meal.

4. Create leftovers!

In today's world, dinner is not made from scratch daily. So on the days you do cook a dinner meal, make extra. The leftovers can be used for lunches in the days ahead. For example, if you cook chicken for dinner, cook a few extra pieces and slice them (or make chicken salad with light mayo) for sandwiches at lunch. When you're making pasta, quinoa, couscous or rice as a side dish for dinner, cook extra to pack as a side dish or combine it with the meat from dinner to make an entrée for lunch.

A Word About Safe Food Packing

Remember . . . when packing a lunch it's essential to keep the food safe to eat by keeping hot foods hot and cold foods cold. I've noticed many parents don't include an ice pack in the lunch bag when packing yogurt, deli-meat sandwiches, string cheese and other foods that need to be kept cold to be safe to eat hours later.

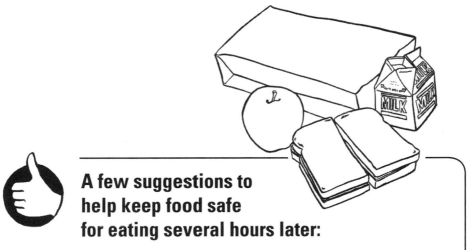

A few suggestions to help keep food safe for eating several hours later:

· Always wash your hands before packing lunch items

· Use a thermos for hot foods if there isn't a microwave available at school

· Use an ice pack even if you don't think the food will spoil

· Freeze foods or drinks the night before. They will thaw by lunch time and serve as a cold pack. Examples include water, 100% juice or yogurt

· Wash out the lunch bag each day

· Include a moist towelette for your child to wash hands before and after eating

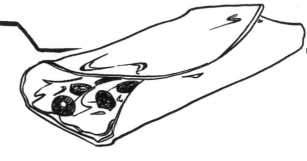

Pizza Wrap

Ingredients :
1 7-inch whole wheat tortilla (taco size)
2 tablespoons spaghetti sauce
10 baby spinach leaves
1 tablespoon chopped fresh basil
¼ cup (1 oz.) shredded part-skim mozzarella

Optional toppings: chopped olives, mushrooms or tomatoes

Preparation :
1. Spread spaghetti sauce evenly over tortilla.
2. Place spinach and basil over sauce.
3. Top with cheese and any other toppings.
4. Microwave on HIGH for 30- 45 seconds or until cheese is melted.
5. Roll tortilla and serve.
Makes 1 serving

If packing in a lunch, let cool 15 minutes, then wrap in foil to refrigerate overnight to pack in a lunch bag with a cold pack.

Note: You can also cut the wrap into rounds and serve as finger food pizza pinwheels.

Nutrition Information per serving :
236 calories, 9g Total Fat, 4g Saturated Fat, 15mg Cholesterol, 534mg Sodium, 26g Carbohydrate, 2g Fiber, 12g Protein

This recipe can be made for lunch at home and eaten warm or it can be made the night before and packed in a school lunch.

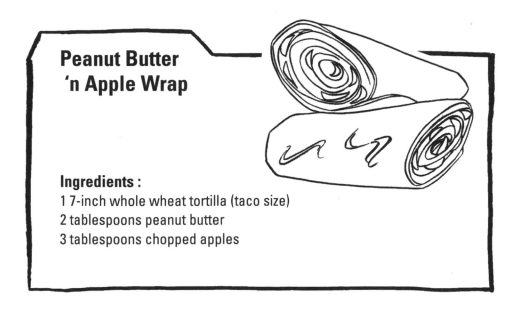

Peanut Butter 'n Apple Wrap

Ingredients :
1 7-inch whole wheat tortilla (taco size)
2 tablespoons peanut butter
3 tablespoons chopped apples

Preparation :
1. Spread peanut butter evenly over tortilla.
2. Place apples 1-2 inches from the edge of the tortilla in a long strip.
3. Roll closest edge of tortilla around apples and continue rolling.
4. Wrap in foil to pack for school lunch or serve immediately.
Makes 1 serving

Nutrition Information per serving :
330 calories, 18g Total Fat, 3g Saturated Fat, 0mg Cholesterol, 493mg Sodium, 35g Carbohydrate, 5.5g Fiber, 12g Protein

Variations: substitute banana slices for the chopped apples; or add 1 tablespoon raisins along with the apples or bananas

Kids love the sweet, crunchiness of the apples in this wrap! And by choosing a whole wheat tortilla instead of a white flour tortilla, you double the fiber, and it counts as a serving of whole grains.

Lunch Box Pasta

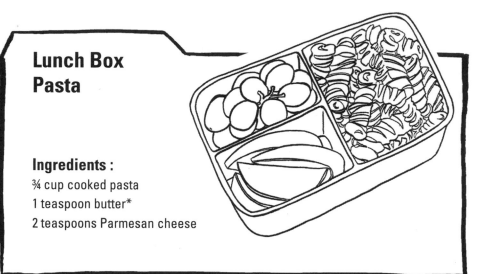

Ingredients :

¾ cup cooked pasta
1 teaspoon butter*
2 teaspoons Parmesan cheese

Preparation :

1. Place pasta in a microwave safe bowl.
2. Spread butter over top of pasta and microwave on HIGH for 45 seconds.
3. Mix melted butter throughout pasta and transfer to a plastic container.
4. Sprinkle with Parmesan cheese, cover with air tight lid and pack for school lunch.
Makes 1 serving

Nutrition Information per serving :

204 calories, 6g Total Fat, 3g Saturated Fat, 14mg Cholesterol,
91mg Sodium, 31g Carbohydrate, 1.5g Fiber, 7g Protein

NutritionTip :

To lower the saturated fat and make this recipe even healthier, use Light butter, which has half the fat and calories of regular butter.

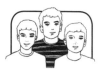

This recipe can be made the night before and refrigerated or put together in the morning to go straight into a lunch bag. When one of my boys was in elementary school, he ate this once or twice a week.

The Bottom Line :

The top 4 lunch entrees Nutrition Experts feed their kids are PB&J sandwich, turkey sandwich, pasta and cheese sandwich. Providing a healthy lunch for your child is essential. By providing a healthy entrée, fruit, vegetable and water or low fat milk (instead of a high fat, high sugar load), your child will be well-fueled, more alert and ready to learn for the rest of the school day!

Your Game Plan :

Three examples that could support your plan are…

1. I will read the Nutrition Facts label before buying cookies for lunch.
2. I will cook extra at dinner to use leftover for lunches.
3. My child and I will decide "school lunch" days at the beginning of the month.

Now that you have some new, healthy ideas for lunch, what will you change about your child's lunch at home and at school?

Healthy Lunch Plan:

1. _____

2. _____

3. _____

Share Your Thoughts . . .

What changes have you made to make lunches healthier for your kids? I would love to hear what was easy about the changes you made? What challenges did you have? Have you noticed any benefits from making the changes? Are there any great tips or ideas you'd like to share?

**Please go to my website: www.400moms.com
or send me an e-mail at Jill@400moms.com
to share your thoughts and comments!**

CHAPTER 5

DINNER

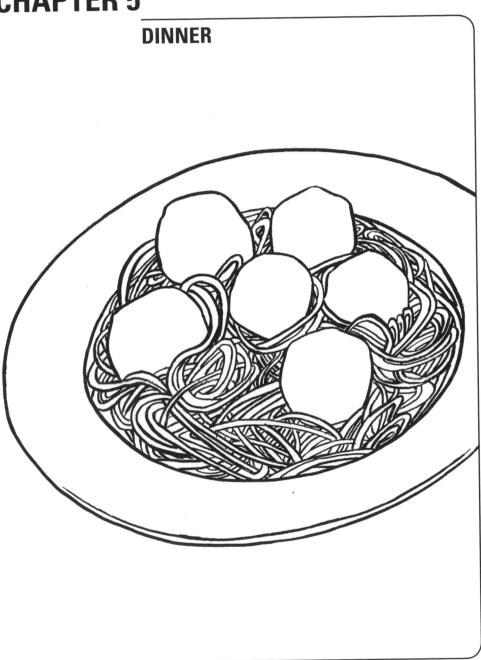

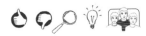

"Mom, What's for Dinner?"

I'm sure I'm not the only parent who is asked this question every night around 5:30pm! In addition to driving to and from after-school activities, helping with homework and taking care of household duties, there's always dinner to fix!

Preparing the dinner meal presents many challenges, including how to get a healthy meal on the table with busy schedules, hungry stomachs and tired bodies. Many Americans have turned to fast food meals and take out dinners to solve their dinner challenges. The National Restaurant Association reports that Americans eat out an average of 4 meals per week, and research shows that Americans now spend 48.9% of their food dollars away from home. Unfortunately, these meals can create new challenges, including too much weight gain, high blood pressure, high cholesterol and poor nutrition.

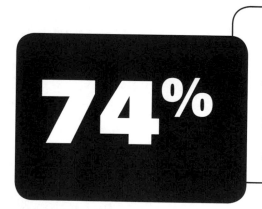

In my survey of Registered Dietitians, 74% reported serving dinner at home *6 or 7 nights per week*.

Another way to look at this statistic is that 74% of Nutrition Experts purchase meals at restaurants or fast food chains *once per week OR LESS* for their families! Why would so many Nutrition Experts be serving almost all dinner meals at home instead of eating out?

Here are just a few of the many benefits of eating at home and eating together as a family:

1. Portion Control

The size of meals served in restaurants is usually **double or triple** the recommended portion size. But once it's in front of us, what do we do? Eat it all! At home you have control over the portion served and by providing the recommended serving size you can help prevent excessive weight gain for you and your kids.

2. Ingredient Control

One of the many problems with restaurant meals is the excessive amount of fat and salt used to prepare the food. By preparing dinner at home you have control over how much oil you use in cooking, how much salad dressing goes on the salad and which side dish to serve. By limiting condiments (i.e. butter, mayonnaise, sour cream, cheese sauce, cream sauce and salad dressing), serving a fruit and vegetable as side dishes and serving milk instead of soda, you have provided an abundance of fiber, calcium and vitamins, instead of an abundance of "empty" calories.

3. Healthy Lifestyle

By controlling the ingredients and portions, the meal you prepare at home will have many more nutrients and much less fat, salt and calories than the meal eaten out. These healthier meals teach your child what foods to include on his plate and can help lower the chances that he will develop diabetes, heart disease and obesity - now and as an adult.

4. Quality Time

Eating together provides an opportunity to talk and connect with your family. Research shows that family dinners 5 or more times per week is associated with lower rates of smoking, drinking and illegal drug use in pre-teens and teens compared to families who eat together 2 or fewer times per week. Another study published in 2011 found that children who share at least 3 family meals together each week are 12% less likely to be overweight and 24% more likely to eat healthy foods.

5. Life Skills

By involving your children in preparing the dinner meal, they're learning valuable self-sufficiency skills. Many kids growing up today lack basic cooking, baking and food preparation skills. Preschoolers can tear lettuce, wash fruit and set the table. Older kids can pour milk, cut some foods and mix ingredients together. Teenagers can dice, chop, bake and boil foods. Working together will get the meal on the table faster and teach healthy eating habits. Involving kids in the preparation of meals creates greater "ownership" of the meal, which leads to greater acceptance of the foods served. In other words, there is less complaining and more eating. Who doesn't want that?

6. Save Money

Restaurant meals frequently cost 2 - 4 times more than a meal prepared at home. So eating at home can save money in short-term food costs and long-term health bills.

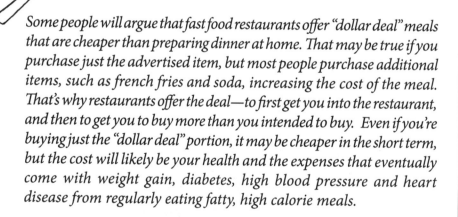

Some people will argue that fast food restaurants offer "dollar deal" meals that are cheaper than preparing dinner at home. That may be true if you purchase just the advertised item, but most people purchase additional items, such as french fries and soda, increasing the cost of the meal. That's why restaurants offer the deal—to first get you into the restaurant, and then to get you to buy more than you intended to buy. Even if you're buying just the "dollar deal" portion, it may be cheaper in the short term, but the cost will likely be your health and the expenses that eventually come with weight gain, diabetes, high blood pressure and heart disease from regularly eating fatty, high calorie meals.

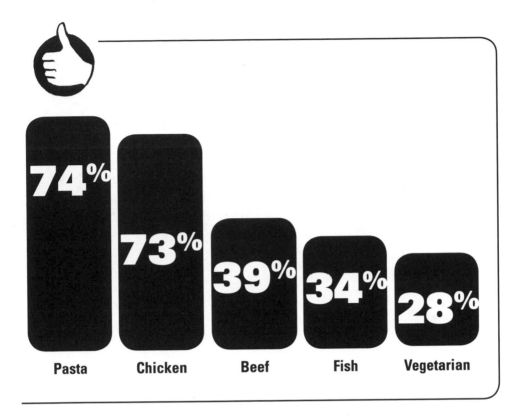

The Top 5 Dinner Entrees Registered Dietitians feed their kids are . . .

#1: **Pasta**

#2: **Chicken - Baked, Grilled or Stir-Fry**

#3: **Ground Beef - Including Meatloaf, Meatballs, Meat Sauce, Hamburgers, Chili**

#4: **Fish - Baked, Grilled or Stir-Fry**

#5: **Vegetarian - Including Beans, Soy Products, Tofu, Cheese Quesadillas, Vegetarian Chili, Vegetarian Lasagna**

When I asked Nutrition Experts to list the most common dinner entrees they serve their kids, the results showed pasta dishes and chicken were by far the most common with almost 3 out of 4 Nutrition Experts listing these two dinners.

Ground beef, fish and vegetarian options (not including pasta) were the next most frequently listed entrees.

It's worth noting that fish and vegetarian options ranked higher than tacos, burritos, pizza and chicken nuggets. What I take from this data is that if fish and vegetarian options rank #4 and #5, then their kids must be eating them!

The Take-Home Message :

If you don't currently serve fish or vegetarian options to your child, it's worth trying them more often!   Your kids may surprise you and like them well enough to replace some of the fast food and frozen dinner options that are higher in fat and sodium.

I'm So Busy. What Do I Do for a Quick Dinner?

Is there a way to balance busy schedules and still make dinner at home each night?

Using quick cooking methods and finding entrees that are quick to prepare can certainly help. I find getting ideas from other parents facing similar challenges is far better than trying to come up with all the ideas myself, so I asked Nutrition Experts to list up to 5 "quick dinner meals" they serve their children. Pasta was by far the winner. Sandwiches, pizza and breakfast foods were equally cited, and burgers of various kinds made the Top-5, but weren't as common.

The Top 5 "Quick" Dinner Meals Served by Nutrition Experts

1 : Pasta
2 : Sandwiches
3 : Pizza
4 : Eggs & Breakfast Foods
5 : Burgers

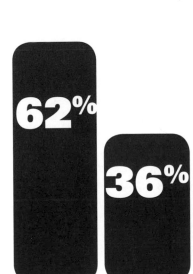
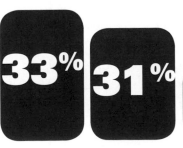

62% — Pasta
36% — Sandwiches
33% — Pizza
31% — Breakfast Foods
13% — Burgers

Top-5 "Quick" Dinner Meals . . .

1 : Pasta

Pasta is an appealing dinner when short on time because cooking time is short and kids love pasta. Although pasta and other "carbs" have gotten a bad rap in the media in recent years, they're actually a **very healthy choice** for your kids and far better than a fast food meal. Another great thing about pasta is that you can make it in a variety of ways, which helps keep kids from getting bored with this quick meal option. Here are a few ways Nutrition Experts serve pasta:

- **Spaghetti with meat sauce or Pasta with meatballs**
  The key to keeping this a healthy choice is to use **extra lean beef.** How do you know if it's extra lean? Check the label for ground beef marked **"93/7", which means it's 93% fat-free and 7% fat.** By choosing extra lean beef you maximize the healthy protein your child gets and minimize the unhealthy fat that's in most cuts of beef.

  As part of my research I attempted to find a frozen beef meatball that met the criteria for a low fat protein choice (10 grams Total Fat/3 oz.), but none of the brands I researched qualified, so making your own meatballs is ideal.

- **Whole Wheat Pasta with marinara sauce**
  Nutrition Experts frequently cited whole wheat spaghetti or pasta with a variety of sauces. The benefit of whole wheat or whole grain noodles is they provide a whole grain serving, while white flour pasta doesn't count as a whole grain and the fiber is more than double in whole grain pastas. For example, whole wheat spaghetti has 6 grams of fiber per cup, while traditional spaghetti has 2 of grams fiber per cup. Give it a try!

- **Macaroni & Cheese**
  This dish can be healthy if you're careful about the brand you buy and how you prepare it. I recommend brands with as few ingredients as possible to minimize the additives and dyes that are common in some brands. For example, Annie's brand macaroni & cheese is made with pasta, real cheese and natural additives. Another very important key to keeping macaroni & cheese healthy is to **use nonfat or 1% milk and no butter when preparing it.** This can be done with any brand of macaroni & cheese. While the macaroni is cooking, mix the milk and powdered cheese together in a separate bowl. When the pasta is cooked and drained, return the hot pasta to the pot, add the cheese sauce and stir well. No butter needed and kids don't notice it missing. *By omitting the butter, you cut out as much as 15 grams of unhealthy fat and 135 calories per one-cup serving!*

- **Pasta with turkey meat sauce or turkey meatballs**
  Most people assume ground turkey is a healthy choice and most of the time it is. However, if there isn't a label telling you how much fat it contains, then it's possible that the skin has been ground in with the meat, in which case it's no longer a healthy choice. So, just like with beef, **look for ground turkey that is labeled "93/7"**, or 93% fat-free and no more than 7% fat. You can also purchase extra lean ground turkey, which is 99% fat free.

There are several brands of frozen turkey meatballs that meet the criteria for a low fat protein choice.

Frozen Meatballs : I recommend turkey meatballs because there are several brands that qualify as a healthy protein choice. When buying frozen turkey meatballs, look for brands that have no more than **10 grams of Total Fat / 3 oz. serving.**

Note: Some brands list the serving size in grams instead of ounces, so the equivalent to 3 oz. is 85-90 grams.

- **Pasta with Parmesan cheese**

  A very simple, quick meal that, when combined with a fruit, vegetable and milk, makes for a well-rounded meal. Although lower in protein than the other pasta options, it's still a healthy choice. You can also provide a protein source on the side, such as string cheese or deli meat rolls if the protein is needed. However, a few "non-meat" or vegetarian meals each week is perfectly healthy.

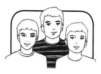 This was a favorite meal for one of my boys when he was 9 years old, and I think he would have eaten it daily if he could! Now that he's a teenager, he prefers the pasta with turkey meatballs for the extra protein.

- **Tortellini or Ravioli with marinara**

  Because these pastas are usually fresh, the cooking time is about half that of dry pastas, so it helps get the meal on the table a little faster. The marinara sauce counts as a vegetable if each serving has at least ½ cup of sauce, so I find it a great way to sneak in a second vegetable. I still serve a fruit and vegetable along with the pasta, so that way my kids get *2 vegetables* and 1 fruit with the meal.

- **Lasagna**

  Homemade lasagna can be a time-consuming meal to prepare, so it doesn't usually make the weekday menu for most families. If there's time on the weekend to make homemade lasagna, be sure to make extra to have as a quick left-over dinner during the week.

  If you're going to buy frozen lasagna, the good news is there are healthy options available, but it will take some careful label-reading to find them.

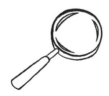 *My recommendation : choose brands that have no more than 10 grams of Total Fat per one-cup serving.*

Be sure to serve one portion size (one cup) and include fruits and vegetables on the plate.

2 : Sandwiches

Sandwiches are what I call an "assemble" dinner that can be prepared with the help of your child. Using whole wheat bread and low fat meat such as ham, turkey or chicken with light mayonnaise, hummus or mustard makes for a healthy entrée portion. Combining the sandwhich with a fruit and vegetable, such as quartered apple and baby carrots completes the meal in less than 10 minutes and provides four different food groups. Add a glass of milk and dinner is complete.

Along with the traditional deli meat sandwiches, Nutrition Experts also serve grilled cheese or grilled turkey & cheese sandwiches. By including the deli meat, you make the grilled cheese sandwich healthier if it substitutes for some of the cheese, which is higher in saturated fat. I suggest lunch meats from the deli counter rather than the pre-packaged and more processed meats.

Many Nutrition Experts also listed "wraps", which can be a nice change from the traditional sandwich and is just as quick to prepare with deli meat or leftover meat from a previous dinner.

By using whole wheat bread for sandwiches your child will get 1-2 whole grain servings, depending on whether she eats a half or whole sandwich. One of my friends, who's also a Registered Dietitian, told me that her kids prefer white bread over whole wheat bread, so they compromise by making what they call a "black and white sandwich": one slice white bread + one slice wheat bread to get at least one whole grain serving and still keep everyone happy.

3 : Pizza

Definitely a favorite in our house! Many Nutrition Experts listed pizza in one form or another: frozen, homemade or takeout as a "quick" meal for their family. I recommend homemade or freshly made pizza over frozen options for two reasons:

#1: Homemade pizza gives you control of *what and how much* goes on your pizza.

#2: Freshly made or takeout pizza is usually less processed and has fewer additives and preservatives than a frozen pizza that was made many months ago.

In terms of quickly getting dinner on the table, homemade pizza can be just as fast as frozen pizza because cooking time is shorter. There are many ways to create a homemade pizza. You can purchase pre-made pizza crust, such as Boboli, or pre-made pizza dough that you roll out yourself.

Another simple version is to use pita bread or a bagel for the crust, and then add pizza sauce and shredded cheese. Pop it under the broiler and pizza is ready in minutes. (See recipe *page 104*) Remember to combine the homemade pizza with a fruit, vegetable and milk and dinner is served!

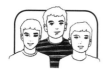 **A word of caution…**to keep pizza from being excessively high in fat, skip the toppings that add more fat on top of the cheese: sausage, ground beef, salami and pepperoni. Instead, choose cheese and add any variety of vegetables on top. As my boys have gotten older, they've discovered that red onion, mushrooms and red pepper make really great vegetable toppings for their pizza.

4 : Eggs & Breakfast Foods

The nice thing about breakfast foods for dinner is that most kids think they're a fun change from typical dinner meals and they can be healthy!

The most common "breakfast for dinner" meals Nutrition Experts serve are (listed in order):

- Eggs
- Pancakes
- Cereal & milk
- French toast
- Waffles

Eggs make a great dinner meal because they're very nutritious and very quick to prepare. Nutrition Experts suggested many different ways they serve them, such as combining scrambled eggs with toast, making omelets, egg sandwiches and breakfast burritos. Eggs do have cholesterol and saturated fat, but can be part of a healthy diet and have over 10 valuable nutrients including high-quality protein, B vitamins, phosphorus, vitamin A & D and choline (a nutrient that is commonly deficient in our diet).

Pancakes, waffles and French toast can also be nutritious choices, unless they're swimming in too much syrup. Pour just enough syrup on top to cover or measure out 1-2 tablespoons of syrup to dip in. Another healthy option is to buy "light" syrup, which has half the sugar and calories and no artificial sweeteners.

Nutrition Tip:

Serve sliced fresh fruit on top of French toast or ¼ cup pureed fruit on pancakes or waffles to replace the syrup and significantly decrease the sugar.

If your kids won't eat a vegetable with "breakfast for dinner", the fruit on top of pancakes or French toast counts as one serving of fruit. I recommend adding a second serving of fruit on the side to replace the missing vegetable serving.

When making French Toast use whole wheat or whole grain bread to make it healthier. When making homemade waffles or pancakes, use pancake mixes with whole grain flour or use ½ white flour and ½ wheat flour in your recipe.

If you don't want to make them from scratch, buy frozen waffles or pancakes made with whole wheat flour.

Look for frozen waffles or pancakes with at least 3 grams of Fiber and no more than 5 grams Total Fat per serving.

5 : Burgers

Just like with meat sauce and meatballs, if you're making burgers from scratch, choose ground beef or ground turkey labeled **"93/7"** to keep the unhealthy fat to a minimum.

When it comes to frozen hamburger patties, well, they're loaded with fat, so I don't recommend them. My advice is to take the extra 5-10 minutes to mix in some spices and make your own from fresh ground meat.

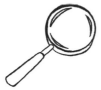

If frozen is your only option, then I recommend frozen turkey burger patties that have **no more than 10 grams of fat per 4 oz. patty** or being really adventurous and trying vegetarian burgers! Veggie burgers are usually about 2 ounces, or half the size of a regular burger. Look for veggie burgers with **no more than 5 grams of fat and at least 10 grams of protein per patty**. If it's a 4 oz. veggie burger, then the nutrition goal is the same as a turkey burger.

In addition to the Top-5 "Quick" Dinner Meals, there are several strategies you can use to make dinner preparation fast enough to eat at home more often.

QUICK & HEALTHY TIPS :

1 : Plan Meals For The Week

Create a dinner calendar where the main entrée stays the same each day of the week - but how you prepare it changes.

EXAMPLE :
Monday = Chicken, Tuesday = Pasta, Wednesday = Lean Ground Beef or Lean Ground Turkey, Thursday = Leftovers, Friday = Fish

Based on your families' schedule and activities, you can decide what types of entrees work best on which nights of the week. Then you can vary how that entrée is made from week to week. For example, on Wednesday you might make hamburgers one week and the next week you might make tacos. This simplifies the grocery shopping, ensures ingredients are available and prevents boredom with the same meals every week.

Another great strategy is Meatless Monday! The name pretty much sums it up: making a dinner meal for your family that doesn't include animal protein. There are many great benefits to this strategy, including:
1. Improving your family's health by starting the week off with a healthy dinner.
2. Helping the environment.
3. Having a dinner plan that is achievable long-term.

Meatless Monday is a non-profit initiative that provides information and recipes on their website: www.meatlessmonday.com where you can learn about the many benefits of a meatless meal and get many great recipes, including over 200 dinner recipes alone. I encourage you to check it out.

You might also substitute a "sandwich night" or "breakfast for dinner" meal instead of leftovers in your weekly plan. Some families include Saturday and Sunday in the meal planning, while others like to leave those meals unplanned depending on weekend activities. You can tailor this meal planning approach to your families' needs, but the most important goal is to simplify meals and shopping so that more dinners are eaten at home.

2 : Create A Standard Shopping List

Take a few minutes to make a grocery list on your computer that includes "staples" (foods you buy regularly), then save it for future use. Next, decide what meals you'll be preparing that week. Print your staples list, circle the staples you need to replenish and write in the additional foods you need that aren't part of your standard list before you go grocery shopping.

The benefits? The bulk of your grocery needs are already written down each time you shop and it saves you time because you just add in a few extras to your main shopping list.

GROCERY LIST:

PRODUCE
- ☐ Lettuce
- ☐ Cucumber
- ☐ Tomatoes
- ☐ Baby Carrots
- ☐ Celery
- ☐ Bell Peppers
- ☐ Broccoli
- ☐ Potatoes
- ☐ Onions
- ☐ Garlic

FRUITS
- ☐ Bananas
- ☐ Apples
- ☐ Oranges
- ☐ Grapes
- ☐ Raisins

MEATS
- ☐ Ground Beef
- ☐ Chicken
- ☐ Ground Turkey
- ☐ Fish
- ☐ Pork

BREADS/GRAINS
- ☐ Bread
- ☐ Rice
- ☐ Pasta
- ☐ Tortillas
- ☐ Crackers
- ☐ Cereals

CANNED FOODS
- ☐ Pears
- ☐ Peaches
- ☐ Applesauce
- ☐ Green Beans
- ☐ Tomatoes
- ☐ Pasta Sauce

BEANS
- ☐ Black
- ☐ Pinto
- ☐ Kidney
- ☐ Garbanzo

CONDIMENTS
- ☐ Light Sour Cream
- ☐ Light Butter
- ☐ Light Cream Cheese
- ☐ Light Salad Dressing
- ☐ Peanut Butter
- ☐ Low-Sugar Jam

DELI
- ☐ Turkey
- ☐ Ham
- ☐ Parmesan Cheese
- ☐ String Cheese

DAIRY
- ☐ Nonfat Milk
- ☐ Eggs
- ☐ Yogurt
- ☐ Cottage Cheese

FROZEN
- ☐ Waffles
- ☐ Light Ice Cream
- ☐ Turkey Meatballs

3 : Create Leftovers

When you're cooking a meal, be sure to make extra! You're already making the meal and it won't take any extra time to make more. Not only that, it will save you preparation and cooking time the rest of the week. Yet one more benefit…it is one of the best ways to save money.

There are so many ways to use leftover chicken, lean beef or pork. Here are a few simple ways to use leftovers:

Chicken noodle soup: Sauté onions, celery and carrots in a small amount of oil; add broth, noodles (dry or leftover) and leftover chicken. Add a few spices and dinner is ready.

Chicken & bean tacos: Quickly sauté some onions and canned roasted chile peppers in a little bit of oil; add leftover chicken, a can of black beans or pinto beans (rinsed and drained); heat through, then spoon the chicken/bean mixture into a corn or flour tortilla and top with chopped lettuce and salsa or tomatoes.

Easy BBQ chicken pizza: Use a premade pizza crust, top with BBQ sauce, chicken, light mozzarella and any veggies your kids will eat. Bake until cheese is melted and dinner is on.

Chicken Pasta Salad (see recipe on *page 102*)

Chicken Fajitas: Sauté onions and sweet peppers in a small amount of oil; add your favorite spices; add chicken and salsa; serve!

Chicken Quesadilla: Using a nonstick pan, place tortilla in heated pan. Sprinkle ½ of tortilla with a 1 oz. of cheese, add chopped chicken. Fold tortilla over and cook until brown and crisp. Flip over and cook other side until crispy. Done!

Chicken & Rice: Combine leftover cooked rice and chopped, cooked chicken in a saucepan; add your favorite spices; heat through and serve.

With all of these leftover ideas, be sure to add a fruit, vegetable and nonfat or low fat milk, to complete the Healthy Plate. (See *page 100*)

Keep in mind that all of the above recipes can be made with beef or pork leftovers. Just be sure to choose the lean cuts of meat.

4 : Use Quick-Cooking Methods

Just about every night one or more of my hungry kids comes into the kitchen and asks, "When will dinner be ready?" There's always a sigh of relief when my answer is "about 10 minutes". If dinner is more than 10 to 15 minutes away, it becomes a sigh of impatience, followed by, "I'm starving!" I understand the need to get dinner on the table ASAP! Some examples of cooking methods that get dinner on the table fast are listed below:

Grilling : Using a gas grill or grill pan for cooking chicken, fish, or meat is much faster than baking because the food is cooked at a higher temperature, so it takes less time.

Stir-frying : Because the pieces of meat are cut up and the cooking temperature is high, this method, like grilling, is fast. There is more preparation time with the chopping, unless you buy the vegetables already chopped or frozen.

Broiling : A great method for cooking fish, chicken breast and hamburgers. It's also great for melting cheese when making homemade pizza.

Assembling : Not an official quick-cooking term, but one I created and believe in! It's great for making dinner from leftovers. For example, you can quickly combine left-over chicken and rice and heat on the stovetop or in the microwave. Or assemble a beef wrap with lettuce, tomatoes and cucumber from leftover grilled steak. By creating a left-over entrée and combining it with a fruit and vegetable, dinner is much healthier and on the table as quickly as the take out meal from the drive-thru.

Re-Heating : Another unofficial cooking term that I made up! It's like assembling in that you quickly combine an entrée with a fruit and vegetable, but different in that you're re-heating a pre-cooked, frozen entrée that you have on hand. For example, most kids love fast food Chicken Nuggets. So instead of going through the drive-thru and buying chicken nuggets, french fries and a soda, you can heat up frozen, pre-cooked chicken nuggets. Although all by themselves these chicken nuggets aren't the healthiest choice, it's much healthier than the fast food option because they're baked (not fried) and when you combine them with a fruit, vegetable and milk, it makes a relatively healthy meal compared to the fast food combination. So it's the best of both worlds: the kids are happy because they get a fast food-like meal and you feel good about making it healthier. Remember to compare brands of the frozen foods to find the option that is lowest in fat.

The Healthy Plate

As you plan and prepare a meal for your child - visualize this model to put together a balanced, nutritious meal for your child

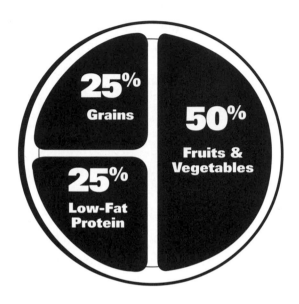

THE HEALTHY PLATE

For many years I've been using this visual of a Healthy Plate to help people understand what portions of each food group they need for a healthy balance. Finally, the USDA has changed the visual they use from the Food Pyramid, which was difficult to understand, to "Choose MyPlate", which is easy to remember and visualize.

Although not all meals will be separated in this way, the idea still works. For example, if you're making hamburgers, they will count as the "Grains" (hamburger bun) and "Protein" (burger) half of the plate. Then the other half of the plate gets filled with a fruit and a vegetable. For example, you might serve a hamburger + sliced oranges + steamed broccoli, creating The Healthy Plate.

One important note : *Over time children adopt the eating habits of their parents, so serving yourself The Healthy Plate is really important if your goal is to encourage healthy eating habits in your child.*

Tasty Tuna Salad

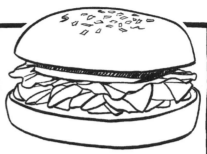

Ingredients :

2 (7 oz.) cans tuna packed in water, drained

1 medium carrot, peeled and grated

1 large stalk celery, diced

1 whole dill pickle, diced

6 tablespoons light sour cream*

2 teaspoons yellow mustard

¼ teaspoon garlic powder

¼ teaspoon black pepper

5 lettuce leaves, washed and dried (optional)

5 tomato slices (optional)

5 Hamburger Buns**

Nutrition Note: By using light sour cream instead of mayonnaise you cut out 100 calories and 12 grams of fat without changing the taste or texture of the recipe!

* * Can substitute whole wheat bread or pita pocket for hamburger bun.

Preparation :

1. In a large bowl, combine tuna, carrot, celery and pickle.
2. Add sour cream, mustard, garlic powder, pepper. Stir until thoroughly mixed.
3. Toast hamburger buns.
4. Place ½ cup tuna on hamburger bun. Top with lettuce and tomato, if desired.
5. Top with other half of bun and serve.

Makes 5 servings

Nutrition Information per serving (tuna salad only) :

122 calories, 2g Total Fat, 1g Saturated Fat, 31mg Cholesterol, 4g Carbohydrate, 557mg Sodium, 1g Fiber, 20g Protein

Nutrition Information per serving (tuna salad with bun) :

292 calories, 4.5g Total Fat, 1g Saturated Fat, 31mg Cholesterol, 35g Carbohydrate, 877mg Sodium, 2g Fiber, 28g Protein

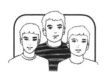

This recipe makes for a very quick dinner! Mix all the ingredients and serve. A few minutes of preparation with no cooking time. You can also pack left-over tuna in a reusable container for a school lunch, along with whole grain crackers (with at least 2 grams Fiber), instead of a bun or bread. My kids really like this tuna served in pita bread.

Chicken Pasta Salad

Ingredients :
8 oz. dry pasta (Fusilli, Penne or Farfalle)
2 medium stalks celery, diced
2 medium carrots, diced
½ medium red bell pepper, diced
3 Tablespoons fresh basil, chopped or 1 1/2 teaspoons dried basil
Black pepper to taste
2 tablespoons olive oil
1/3 cup Light Italian salad dressing
1 ½ cups cooked chicken, diced
3 tablespoons Parmesan cheese

Preparation :
1. Cook pasta according to package directions, omitting fat.
2. While pasta is cooking, combine celery, carrots, red pepper in a large bowl.
3. When pasta is cooked, rinse under cold water, add to vegetable mixture.
4. Add remaining ingredients and mix well to coat.
5. Refrigerate for at least 1 hour before serving.
Makes 8 servings

Nutrition Information per serving :
202 calories, 6g Total Fat, 1g Saturated Fat, 24mg Cholesterol, 237mg Sodium, 24g Carbohydrate, 2g Fiber, 13g Protein

Nutrition Note :
Substitute whole wheat pasta for traditional pasta to increase the fiber and get a serving of whole grains!

This recipe can be made in advance so it's ready to serve with a fruit and vegetable after a busy day. Be sure to make extra because the left-overs make a great lunch for school or work.

Pizza Quesadilla

Ingredients :
2 10-inch (burrito size) whole wheat tortillas
¼ cup spaghetti sauce
½ cup baby spinach leaves
2 tablespoons fresh basil (optional)
½ cup shredded part-skim mozzarella

Optional toppings:
chopped olives
or mushrooms

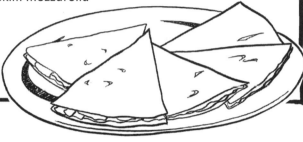

Preparation :
1. Spread spaghetti sauce evenly over tortilla.
2. Place spinach and basil on top of sauce.
3. Sprinkle with cheese and any other toppings. Place 2nd tortilla on top.
4. Spray a nonstick pan with oil. Heat pan over medium-high heat for one minute, then add quesadilla.
5. Cook 2-3 minutes or until one side of tortilla is brown.
   Flip and continue cooking until bottom tortilla is brown and crispy.
6. Remove from pan and cool 1-2 minutes, then cut into 6 triangles.
Makes 2 servings

Nutrition Information per serving (3 triangles) :
335 calories, 12g Total Fat, 4.5g Saturated Fat, 15mg Cholesterol,
745mg Sodium, 43g Carbohydrate, 2.5g Fiber, 14g Protein

This recipe takes about 5 minutes to make and combined with a fruit and vegetable provides 4 food groups in one meal for your child. It's a modified version of the Pizza Wrap recipe on *page 76* in Chapter 4 and is best served warm. Now that my boys are old enough to prepare meals themselves, they make this recipe frequently for lunch on the weekend or dinner anytime. My boys like this recipe as much as a traditional quesadilla.

Pizza Bagel

Ingredients :
1 medium plain or sesame bagel
3 tablespoons spaghetti sauce
2 tablespoons fresh basil or 1 teaspoon dried basil (optional)
½ cup shredded part-skim mozzarella

Optional toppings: chopped olives, mushrooms or spinach

Preparation :
1. Slice bagel in half and spread spaghetti sauce evenly over each half.
2. Sprinkle basil on top of sauce.
3. Layer with cheese and any other toppings.
4. Place bagels on a foil-lined baking sheet. Broil in oven, just until cheese melts, about 2 minutes. Watch carefully to prevent burning.
5. Remove from oven and cool 1-2 minutes, then serve.
6. For younger children, cut into quarters.
Makes 1-2 servings

Nutrition Information per serving (3 triangles):
240 calories, 7g Total Fat, 3g Saturated Fat, 15mg Cholesterol, 31g Carbohydrate, 503mg Sodium, 1.5g Fiber, 13g Protein

Variation :
Substitute pita bread for the bagel.

This recipe is a variation of the Pizza Quesadilla and takes only a few minutes to make and cook.

The Bottom Line :

The top 4 quick dinner meals nutrition experts feed their kids are pasta, sandwiches, pizza and breakfast foods. Despite busy schedules, providing healthy dinners at home is feasible and can be as fast as takeout meals when a few meal planning strategies and quick cooking methods are in place.

Your Game Plan :

Three examples that could support your plan are...

1. I will try the quick dinner ideas
2. I will make a "staples" grocery list so I have the ingredients to make dinner at home.
3. I will buy frozen vegetables and baby carrots so I'm sure to have enough vegetables to serve at dinner every night.

After reading this chapter, what will you change so your family eats at home more often? How will you make dinners for your child healthier?

The Changes I Will Make To Our Dinner Habits :

1. _____

2. _____

3. _____

Share Your Thoughts . . .

What changes have you made to make dinner healthier for your kids? What you are doing differently to help your family eat at home more often? Have you noticed any benefits from making the changes? What favorite quick & easy recipes are you using? Are there any great tips or ideas you'd like to share?

**Please go to my website: www.400moms.com
or send me an e-mail at Jill@400moms.com
to share your thoughts and comments!**

CHAPTER 6

PRODUCE POWER!

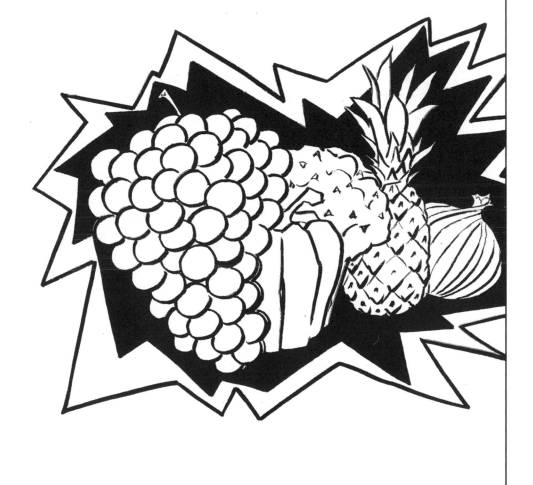

Produce Power!

How many servings of fruit & vegetables does your child need each day? Most parents don't know the answer, and the amount changes as your child grows. Starting in 2003 the "5-A-Day" campaign encouraged Americans to eat a total of 5 servings of fruits and vegetables daily.

Then in 2005 the recommendations changed from "servings" to "cups" and the recommended amount of fruits and vegetables *increased*. Unfortunately, most kids and adults aren't even eating 5 servings each day, let alone more!

In June 2011 the USDA changed its graphics and messaging from "The Food Pyramid" to "Choose MyPlate". The only real change that occurred was that the Meat & Beans group changed its name to the Protein group. Everything else remains the same, including the recommended servings for each food group.

The chart below shows how many fruits and vegetables your child needs based on age and moderate activity:

	2-3 years	4-8 years	9-13 years	14-18 years
Fruit Servings	1 cup	1 ½ cups	1 ½ cups	2 cups*
Vegetable Servings	1 ½ cups	2 cups	3 cups*	3 ½ cups*

Vegetable servings are 1/2 cup less for girls.

Many parents respond to these recommendations with, "1½ cups of vegetables, you've got to be kidding! I can't get Suzie to eat any vegetables, let alone 1½ cups. I've quit trying." I hope you aren't this frustrated, but if you are, keep reading! There may be ideas and strategies you haven't thought of or tried that can help get your child eating more fruits and vegetables.

The recommended servings are difficult to achieve for sure. Many Nutrition Experts aren't reaching the recommendations for their kids!

The results of my survey showed that only 32% of Registered Dietitians offer their kids 3 or more servings (about 1½ cups) of vegetables per day, while 88% of Registered Dietitians serve their kids 2 or more fruits daily (about 1 to 2 cups). Although many Nutrition Experts meet the serving recommendations for kids 2 to 3 years old, these results show how challenging it is to achieve the recommendations as kids get older and servings increase. But with all the health benefits from eating fruits and vegetables, I encourage you to aim for *serving at least 5 total fruits and vegetables each day*.

Here are just a few of the short-term and long-term benefits your child gets from eating fruits and vegetables :

Vitamins & minerals : important for maintaining healthy bones, healthy eyes and strong immunity. They help all systems in your body work at their best.

Fiber : helps fill you up and keeps digestion working smoothly.

Disease risk : can help reduce the risk of heart disease, high blood pressure, Type 2 Diabetes and some cancers.

Low calorie cost : naturally low in calories, yet high in nutrients, which helps us manage weight.

Just for fun, I asked Registered Dietitians what are their kids 3 favorite fruits and vegetables?

FRUITS		VEGETABLES	
Apples	48%	Carrots	45%
Berries	42%	Broccoli	42%
Bananas	32%	Corn	24%
Grapes	24%	Green Beans	22%
Melon	18%	Salad	17%

Would your child agree with these favorites?

I suggest you ask your child what are his or her top 3 choices for fruits and vegetables. That way you know which options to always have available, while mixing in other choices for variety and "re-trying" opportunities (read more about "re-trying" later in this chapter).

Important Note:

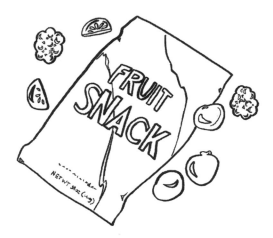

Fruit Snacks are not a fruit serving!

Many packaged fruit snacks, fruit drinks and other snacks advertise *"made with real fruit"* on their labels. Why? To get parents to buy them, thinking they're healthy! It's really just a marketing ploy. If you read the ingredient list you'll see they contain sugar, other sweeteners, artificial flavors and dyes. For example, here are the ingredients for several popular brands:

Welch's Fruit Snacks "Made with Real Fruit"
Ingredients: Juice from concentrates (grape, pear, peach, pineapple), **corn syrup, sugar**, modified cornstarch, fruit purees (strawberry, orange, raspberry, grape), natural and artificial flavors, Red 40, Yellow 5, Blue 1.

Betty Crocker Fruit by the Foot
Ingredients: Pears from concentrate, **sugar**, maltodextrin, **corn syrup**, partially hydrogenated cottonseed oil, Red 40, Yellow 5, Blue 1.

Betty Crocker Fruit Gushers
Ingredients: Pears from concentrate, **dried corn syrup, corn syrup**, modified cornstarch, **fructose**, grape juice from concentrate, Red 40, Blue 1, Yellow 5.

From what I'm reading on these labels, there's not a whole lot of fruit, but plenty of sugar and juice concentrate in these products. They're just glorified candy.

There are a few options available that are made of all fruit, often referred to as "fruit leathers" or "fruit strips", that can count toward daily fruit servings, though not an ideal option.

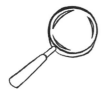

What to look for. . .

As an alternative to fruit snacks,
look for fruit strips that have

fruit as the main ingredient
no juice or juice concentrate
no artificial flavors or dyes.

A few brands to look for include:
- Trader Joe's Fiberful Handmade Dried Fruit Bar
- Trader Joe's Handmade 100% Dried Fruit Bar
- Stretch Island Fruit Company Original Fruit Strips

The ingredients in these brands are dried fruits, fruit puree concentrates and ascorbic acid (vitamin C) or lemon juice as a preservative. No juice, no sugar and no artificial colors or dyes.

What counts as a fruit serving?

For most brands, 2 fruit strips count as the equivalent of ½ cup of fruit. The goal is to get **at least 2 grams of fiber and no more than 100 calories.** For example, a Trader Joe's Handmade 100% Dried Fruit Bar contains 1.5 grams fiber and 50 calories, so if your child eats *two* fruit strips it would meet the equivalent for ½ cup fruit because the strips would provide 3 grams of fiber and 100 calories.

I don't encourage fruit strips on a regular basis. Actual dried fruit (mango, raisins, apricots, etc.) is much better. However, it is healthier than dessert, so it does make a nice dessert substitute.

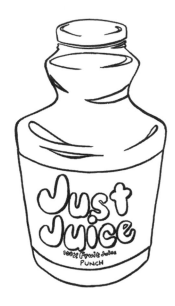

Parents frequently ask, "Is it ok to give my child juice?"

It's true that some juices are a good source of Vitamin C, but so are many other fruits and vegetables, which are not only rich in Vitamin C, but also in fiber and many other valuable nutrients that juices don't offer. So I created a list of alternatives to juice that are a good source of Vitamin C (see next page).

However, there are two exceptions when juice may be a worthwhile choice. If your child is an athlete and has trouble getting enough calories (and is drinking 3-4 cups of milk per day) or your child is in a very picky phase and is refusing ALL fruits and vegetables. In these two situations, some juice may be appropriate, but for most children, juice should be limited.

The whole food is always best; however, if you're going to serve juice, I recommend the following:

1. **Make it 100% juice (make sure there are no added sugars in the ingredient list).**
2. **Dilute juice with 50% water for toddlers and preschoolers.**
3. **Serve ½ cup or less per day.**
4. **Don't serve juice every day.**

Jill's Best Picks :
Vitamin C-Rich Choices

Fruits	Vegetables
Apricots	Bell peppers (red, green, yellow, orange)
Blackberries	Broccoli
Cantaloupe	Brussel Sprouts
Grapefruit	Cabbage
Guava	Cauliflower
Kiwifruit	Potato
Honeydew Melon	Spinach
Orange	Summer Squash
Papaya	Sweet Potato
Pineapple	Tomato
Raspberries	
Strawberries	
Tangerines	
Watermelon	

113

So how do you get your kids to eat more fruits and vegetables, when all they want is chicken nuggets and french fries?

 # 1 : Start early - If you have a toddler start now. By offering a toddler many types of foods, the odds are greater that she will eat a variety of foods as she grows older. Children's food preferences and food-intake patterns are shaped largely by the foods parents make available to children and by persistence in presenting a food that initially is rejected.

 # 2 : Try, try again! - The good news is, not all is lost if your child is past the toddler age. If your child is given repeated opportunities to try new foods, they are more likely to eventually eat those foods. Which means you may have to offer a small portion of a vegetable (i.e. 3 or 4 green beans) 10-15 times before your child will eat it. Thus, the motto "**TRY, TRY AGAIN!**" is an important reminder when you're feeling frustrated by your child's rejection of vegetables or other foods.

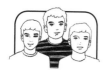 My personal experience has been that kids go through phases where an accepted food is suddenly being rejected and then months or sometimes years later, they return to liking that particular food again. For example, one of my boys *loved* green beans when he was about 3 years old. Then, suddenly, out of nowhere he started refusing to eat them. I gave them a break for a few months, then began "re-trying" them every once in a while. It took about 2 years, but eventually he returned to eating green beans without a fuss.

Frustrating, I know, but my advice is to keep serving the rejected food periodically and eventually your child is likely to return to eating it. If, on the other hand, you give up and stop serving that food, your child loses the opportunity to rediscover liking it!

 # 3 : Walk the Walk - Toddlers and preschoolers pay a lot of attention to what their parents eat. So you can have a big influence on what your kids like to eat by modeling eating healthy foods yourself. By showing your child that you eat and enjoy fruits and vegetables, you are helping increase the chances that he, too, will eat them. The opposite also holds true… if you rarely serve vegetables on your plate or rarely eat fruit, don't be surprised if your child develops the same eating habits.

4 : Offer the Rainbow

By offering a variety of colors of fruits and vegetables, you can help prevent boredom with food choices and be sure your child gets the wide variety of vitamins and nutrients her body needs.

When preparing a meal for your child, ask yourself, "How many colors are on the plate?" Try to offer different colors at different meals. The more colors throughout the day, the better.

Here are a few examples of fruits and vegetables by color:

Purple/Blue	Green	White	Yellow/Orange	Red
Blueberries	Pears	Bananas	Oranges	Cherries
Plums	Broccoli	White Nectarines	Apricots	Strawberries
Grapes	Green beans	Jicama	Pineapple	Watermelon
Eggplant	Green apples	Cauliflower	Carrots	Red apples
Blackberries	Kiwifruit	Potatoes	Butternut Squash	Beets
Raisins	Snow Peas	Mushrooms	Corn	Tomatoes
	Lettuce	Onions	Sweet Potatoes	Red peppers
	Spinach			Tomato Sauce

Take a minute to circle at least 3 choices in each color group that you can serve to your child in the next week or two.

Talk with your child about the many colors of fruits and vegetables and ask which ones are her favorites. The different colors of produce offer different substances (vitamins, minerals, antioxidants, carotenoids, phytochemicals and bioflavonoids to name a few) that provide great health benefits for the long-term :

Purple/Blue : Helps slow aging, improves memory, healthy urinary tract and may lower cancer risk.

Green : Helps eyesight, bones and teeth, and may lower cancer risk.

White : Helps with heart health and may lower cancer risk.

Yellow/Orange : Helps eyesight, immune system, heart and may lower cancer risk.

Red : Helps with heart health, blood vessels, improving memory and may lower cancer risk.

A key principle I emphasize with parents is this:

Your job as the parent is to teach your child about healthy eating (even if the healthy foods are rejected)

The theory behind this principle is that if kids are consistently exposed to healthy eating, they are more likely to adopt healthy eating habits as they get older.

I know many examples of children who were "picky eaters" at a young age, but eventually developed healthy eating habits as they got older. By consistently providing variety and healthy choices, these habits are frequently adopted by kids… eventually.

A true story and perfect example of this is the son of my good friend and neighbor, Lisa. As her children were growing up, she and her husband modeled healthy eating and served healthy meals to their 3 kids. But despite Lisa's best efforts, her son "hated vegetables", loved Fast Food and soda and took every opportunity to complain about fruits and vegetables. It wasn't until *he was in his late 20's* that he began to change his ways. Because his parents had taught him what a healthy plate looked like, he had the skills and knowledge to change his eating habits when he was ready and motivated to do so.

There are three take home messages here:
- Try, try again!
- Model healthy eating
- Provide A Healthy Plate at mealtimes (see *page 104*)

Even though your main job is to *provide the fruits and vegetables*, I know most parents also want their kids to *eat them*! So I asked Registered Dietitians what strategies they use to get *their* kids to eat fruits and vegetables.

In the next chapter, I talk about the many ideas and strategies that Nutrition Experts use that you can try too! In the meantime, I've included a few kid-tested recipes on the next few pages that might get your kids eating fruits and vegetables without a lot of convincing needed!

Apple-Carrot Salad w/ Raisins

Ingredients :
2 cups store-bought shredded carrots
1 large Granny Smith apple, cored and diced
½ cup raisins
1 tablespoon fresh lemon juice
½ cup nonfat vanilla yogurt
½ teaspoon ground cinnamon or to taste (optional)

Preparation :
1. Combine carrots, apple, raisins and lemon juice. Stir well.
2. Add yogurt and stir again.
3. Sprinkle with cinnamon and serve.
Makes 7 ½-cup servings

Nutrition Information per ½-cup serving :
74 calories, 0g Total Fat, 0g Saturated Fat, 0mg Cholesterol, 34mg Sodium, 18g Carbohydrate, 2g Fiber, 1.5g Protein

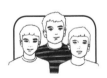 Here's a great way to get your kids eating fruits and vegetables, all in one dish. It's important to note that I buy the carrots already shredded (you can find them in the refrigerated produce section of your grocery store) because it saves a lot of preparation time and these carrots make the salad crunchy, not mushy.

All 3 of my boys love this recipe!

Sweet Broccoli Slaw

Ingredients :
2 cups broccoli slaw
1 cup store-bought shredded carrots
1 large Granny Smith apple, cored and diced
½ cup raisins
1 tablespoon fresh lemon juice
½ cup nonfat vanilla yogurt
½ teaspoon ground cinnamon or to taste (optional)

Preparation :
1. Combine broccoli slaw, carrots, apple, raisins and lemon juice. Stir well.
2. Add yogurt and stir again.
3. Sprinkle with cinnamon and serve.
Makes 10 ½-cup servings

Nutrition Information per ½-cup serving :
54 calories, 0g Total Fat, 0g Saturated Fat, 0mg Cholesterol, 23mg Sodium, 13g Carbohydrate, 2g Fiber, 1.5g Protein

Never heard of Broccoli Slaw? It's a great source of Vitamin A and C and is available prepackaged in the produce section of your grocery store. It's shredded stems of broccoli. Many kids like it better than the florets and it works great in salads! Here's another great way to get your kids to eat fruits and vegetables in one dish! Again, buying the carrots already shredded saves time and adds crunchiness that makes all the difference.

Asian Broccoli Slaw

Ingredients :
2 cups broccoli slaw
2 cups store-bought shredded carrots
1 tablespoon fresh lemon juice
3 tablespoons slivered almonds
3 tablespoons Newman's Own low fat Sesame Ginger salad dressing

Preparation :
1. Combine broccoli slaw, carrots, lemon juice and almonds in a large bowl. Stir well.
2. Add sesame dressing and mix to coat, then serve.

Makes 10 ½-cup servings

Nutrition Information per serving :
46 Calories, 2g Total Fat, 0g Saturated Fat, 0mg Cholesterol, 101mg Sodium, 6g Carbohydrate, 2g Fiber, 1.5g Protein

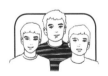

This version of broccoli slaw is less sweet, very crunchy and all vegetables. It's quick to prepare, and is very popular in my family. You can substitute shredded cabbage for the broccoli slaw to add variety. My kids like that too, but not as much as the broccoli slaw. Sometimes I chop up left-over cooked chicken breast and add it to this salad. My teenage boys like the extra protein.

A Word of Caution :

While you are trying to increase the amount of fruits and vegetables your child eats, it can be easy to lose sight of the bigger picture, which is teaching healthy habits.

Please keep these healthy habits in mind:

· Don't force your child to "clean your plate"

· Avoid power struggles about food and meals

· Parent's job: provide the fruits and vegetables

· Child's job: decide what and how much to eat

· Parent's job: be a role model by eating fruits & vegetables yourself

· Keep mealtimes enjoyable and relaxed

If you're worried that your child is an excessively picky eater and is not getting many of the nutrients he or she needs, consider offering a chewable multi-vitamin and talk to your Pediatrician or a Registered Dietitian to obtain more specific, individualized recommendations.

The Bottom Line :

Your job as the parent is to *provide* the recommended amounts of fruits and vegetables each day. It's your child's job to decide how much of them to eat. By providing the fruits and vegetables, you're teaching your child healthy eating habits for a lifetime. This approach can have the added bonus of decreasing food battles, keeping mealtime positive family time.

Your Game Plan :

Three examples that could support your plan are...

1. I will keep dried fruit and canned fruit on hand in my cupboard.
2. I will serve fruit first at snack time.
3. I will have my child choose the fruit or vegetable option for dinner.

What will you do to make sure you provide the recommended amount of fruits and vegetables for your child? Are there some recipes you might try? Could a fruit or vegetable be included more often at meals or snack times?

1. _____

2. _____

3. _____

Share Your Thoughts . . .

I would love to hear what strategies you've found helpful to get your kids to eat more fruits and vegetables. Are there any great tips or ideas you'd like to share?

Please go to my website: www.**400moms.com** or send me an e-mail at <u>Jill@400moms.com</u> to share your thoughts and comments!

CHAPTER 7

WINNING WITH VEGETABLES!

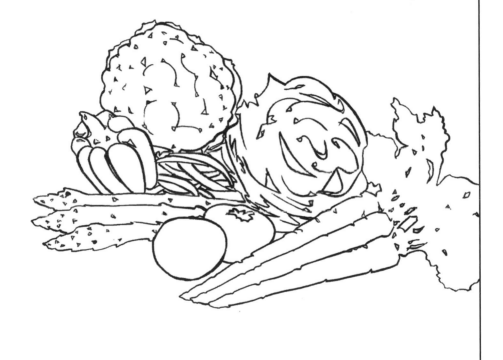

Winning With Vegetables!

Meal time can be a time for power struggles and a "test of wills" for many families, especially when it comes to getting your child to eat vegetables! If you have multiple children, you've probably experienced the same thing I have: each child has different likes and dislikes and the amount of struggle it takes to get them to eat healthy food varies a lot.

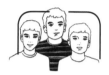 Since the age of 2, my oldest son has always liked trying new foods. My middle son, on the other hand, would *look* at a food on his plate and say, "I don't like that!" My youngest son falls somewhere in between. Depending on his mood, he will like the food one day and reject it the next day.

The good news is that as they've moved into their tween and teen years, my boys are all very willing to try new foods and, frequently, look forward to trying the new recipes their Dad makes.

Our deal is that I cook dinner meals during the week and he cooks on the weekend. I always make sure he prepares extra so I can use the left-overs for quick, healthy meals during the week. And the truth is my husband is a better cook than I am, so his meals make great left-overs.

We've gotten to the point where I no longer need strategies to get my boys to eat vegetables. And very rarely do I have to remind them to "eat your vegetables". I believe it's mostly because of the strategies I used over the years and being consistent with those strategies.

Many of my strategies (I learned through my survey) are used by other Nutrition Experts too. Their suggestions and many more will be shared in this chapter.

Why Is It Kids Don't Like Vegetables?

There are some theories, including research showing that some kids have a gene that influences whether they are sensitive to bitter tastes. Kids who have this gene may be more likely to dislike bitter foods, including vegetables such as broccoli, cabbage, spinach, cucumber and olives. The interesting part of this study was that the mothers who had this same gene did not dislike the bitter vegetables they tasted in the study. So it's possible that we "outgrow" this sensitivity. That's good news and support for continuing to serve vegetables to kids who don't like them because we don't know when they might "outgrow" their sensitivity to bitter tastes and start eating more vegetables.

Another solution is to serve sweeter vegetables more often (carrots, beets, sweet potato) and to try a frozen version (frozen broccoli) or a baby version (baby spinach), which are often less bitter.

Other thoughts and opinions include the possibility that young children's taste buds are more sensitive to sweet foods and as they get older their taste buds change, making vegetables more appealing.

There's also the influence of Mom and Dad. If one or both parents don't like vegetables, and, therefore, don't regularly serve vegetables or have them on their plate, then their kids will likely follow in their footsteps, disliking vegetables, too.

Regardless of *why* your child might dislike vegetables, the bottom line is: **keep serving them!** Why? Because your child learns what a healthy plate looks like, and with time is more likely to broaden the vegetables he or she is willing to eat.

Getting Kids to Eat Their Fruits and Vegetables

Although it's much less common, some parents struggle to get their child to eat fruit or to get them to eat more than the same 2 or 3 fruits all year long. I'll spend a little time talking about strategies to encourage more fruit, but most of the chapter will focus on getting your child to eat vegetables.

There are opposing beliefs about just what parents should or shouldn't do to get their kids to eat healthy foods, including vegetables. The opinions vary from the "No Options" approach to "Serve it and Say No More" approach and everything in between.

No Options

The "No Options" approach involves serving the child a meal or snack and that is what they get. No choices, no substitutions; and there is no other food served until the next meal or snack.

Serve It and Say No More

The "Serve it and Say No More" approach is providing a healthy meal or snack and letting the child decide what and how much to eat, even if it means leaving all the fruits and vegetables behind on the plate. Then there are strategies, such as begging, bribing and rewarding, which I don't recommend.

Through my survey, I asked Registered Dietitians to list 2 to 4 strategies they use to get their kids to eat fruits and vegetables. They provided many great ideas. I'll share the most common strategies and ideas reported so you can decide what to try with your family.

The following "Strategies" are kind of like a Family Rule or approach Nutrition Experts frequently mentioned using with their kids. I've also compiled ideas Nutrition Experts listed that are specific *action steps,* or suggestions, you can use on a daily basis to encourage your child to eat more vegetables.

STRATEGY # 1 :
THE "BITE" RULE

No, I'm not talking about kids biting each other, though I remember that age and phase. Glad we're past it! Instead, I'm referring to the idea that whenever your child is struggling to eat a certain food on his plate, whether it's a new food or a food he doesn't like at the moment, you can have a rule about how many bites he needs to eat.

For some Nutrition Experts, the rule is "one bite", while others specified "two bites" or "three bites". You decide what number of bites works for you. But it goes something like this:

> Timmy says, *"Eeeww, I don't like that green stuff."*

> Mom matter-of-factly answers, *"I want you to try one bite of the asparagus. If you don't like it, you don't have to eat any more."*

You may have to repeat yourself a couple of times. Then once he tries it (and probably says "eeewww, yuk!"), you enthusiastically say, "Thanks for trying it!" and you're done. End of conversation. If he likes it, well, that will be a bonus and one more vegetable you can serve.

Over time "try one bite" encourages your child to try new foods without the pressure of having to eat it all.

As I mentioned in a previous chapter, it can take 10 or more attempts of trying a new food before a child accepts it, so remember the slogan, **"Try, Try Again".**

By using The "Bite" Rule, you minimize the stress around a new food on the plate, yet give your child an opportunity to see if she likes it. This strategy has worked really well with my kids and I believe has expanded the fruits and vegetables they eat because sometimes they have been surprised to find out that they actually liked it! Artichokes and grilled asparagus are two perfect examples.

Along with The "Bite" Rule, several Nutrition Experts commented that they serve a small portion when they introduce a new food to their child. This helps the child feel less overwhelmed or intimidated by having to try something different.

Some Nutritionists also stated that they serve smaller portions of the fruits and vegetables their kids don't like as much and larger portions of the ones they like better. This portion concept can work in two ways. First, if your child likes carrots better than broccoli, then you can serve *a larger number* of carrots than broccoli florets, and secondly, you can serve carrots *more often* than you serve broccoli. For parents who are concerned about wasting food, this strategy helps address that issue by keeping the potentially uneaten portion small. By serving 2 or 3 broccoli florets, you're still teaching what should be on a healthy plate without creating a lot of waste.

Finally, keep in mind that "take one bite" can be a useful strategy, but many Dietitians also commented that they don't "force the issue" around eating any certain foods or amount of food.

If a strategy is creating excessive stress or is a control battle, it becomes counter-productive. Arguing over "one bite" is not beneficial and my suggestion is to let it go. Then, the next time there is a disliked food use the "take one bite" strategy again. Over time, your child will get used to the approach and will be more likely to try it.

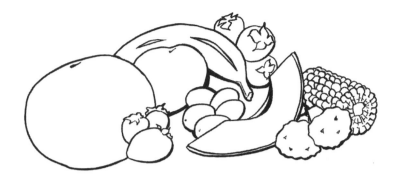

STRATEGY # 2 :
"5-A-DAY EVERYDAY"

As I mentioned in Chapter 6, the goal of the "5-A-Day" campaign in 2003 was to encourage Americans to eat a total of 5 servings of fruits and vegetables daily. Even though the "5-A-Day" concept wasn't clear about how much was in a serving, I find people know and remember the goal of "5-A-Day" much more often than they know how many cups of fruits and vegetables they're supposed to be eating each day.

I believe the 5-a-day goal for the whole family is a really great place to start! As a Mom, I think it's much easier to keep track of the number of fruits and vegetables I've served my kids, rather than focus on the number of cups. I figure if I can serve a total of 5 or more fruits and vegetables in the day (even if the total cups don't quite match what is recommended), then I'm doing a really great job.

If you want to know exactly how many cups of fruits and vegetables your child needs, go to www.choosemyplate.org

At the home page, click on MyPlate. You can choose fruits or vegetables and "how much is needed" and a chart will provide specific servings based on your child's age, gender and activity level.

What's in a cup?

Here are several examples of fruits and vegetables that equal a ½ cup or 1 cup serving:

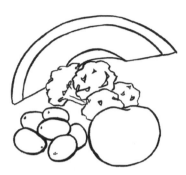 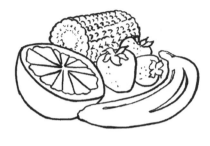

1/2 CUP
5 Broccoli Florets
1 Cantaloupe Wedge
16 Grapes
1 Large Plum

1 CUP
1 Large Banana
1 Medium Grapefruit
8 Large Strawberries
1 Medium Potato or Sweet Potato
12 Baby Carrots
1 Large Ear of Corn

When I see 3 ½ cups of vegetables for my 13-year-old son, my initial reaction is, "Whew, that's a lot of vegetables. How will I ever get him to eat all those vegetables without a big battle?" Do you ever feel defeated before you've even started? That's another reason why I like using the "5-A-Day" approach. It's doable and still teaches your children the importance of choosing fruits and vegetables several times a day, even if the number of fruits is greater than vegetables.

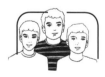 I have to admit, my 13-year old doesn't eat 3 ½ cups of vegetables every day. My approach is to serve a fruit at all 3 meals, have my child choose a fruit or vegetable as part of his afternoon snack and serve 1 to 2 vegetables at dinner. That adds up to 5 to 6 servings for the day and keeps him in the habit of choosing fruits and vegetables.

Always Available

The good news is Nutrition Experts had many comments about what helps their kids get "5-A-Day". The most common suggestion was to have fruits and vegetables "always available".

So what exactly does that mean? It can mean buying enough produce when you go grocery shopping so you don't run out of fruits and vegetables before your next shopping trip. That means planning and purchasing according to how often you plan to shop. For example, if your goal is to go to the grocery store once per week, and you have a family of four, then you will need to buy enough fruits and vegetables to make at least *140 servings*, if the whole family is going to reach the "5-a-Day" goal.

Most of us don't think in these terms when we're in the produce aisle, but your family would be eating 20 fruit and vegetable servings per day (5 servings X 4 people) for 7 days. You may need a few less servings than this if your children are less than 8 years old, since their serving sizes are smaller. It may take some trial and error to find the right amount to purchase, but with time you can accurately estimate how much to purchase depending on how often you go to the grocery store. These fruit and vegetable servings don't have to be all fresh choices either. I recommend having dried fruit, canned fruits and vegetables and frozen options available as well. That way you have back up options if you run out of fresh choices before you get to the grocery store again.

"Always available" can also mean having fruits and vegetables *accessible*.

Here are several examples Nutrition Experts stated:
- "I always keep a bowl of fruit on the kitchen table"
- "We have fruit on the kitchen counter"
- "I put a vegetable plate out before dinner"
- "Fruit is always visible"
- "I keep cut up vegetables in the refrigerator"
- "I make them easy to grab-and-go"
- "Cut up vegetables are out while I'm making dinner"
- "I keep several types of fruit already washed and ready to grab"

Healthy Foods First

Another method Nutrition Experts use to encourage their kids to eat fruits and vegetables is to require "Healthy Foods First" before having other snacks or sweets.

This can be implemented at each meal or for the whole day. For example, at dinner you can have a rule that the fruit and vegetable on the plate need to be eaten before having dessert after dinner.

A similar method stated was **"no sweets or desserts until 5-A-Day has been accomplished"**. So this would apply to the whole day. In order to have dessert or sweets, 5 servings of fruits and vegetables would be eaten first. One benefit to this approach is that by the time fruits and vegetables are eaten, desserts or sweets would most likely be limited to once a day, after the dinner meal.

Fruits and Vegetables Only

Another healthy food first suggestion was to provide fruits and vegetables as the only snack options between meals. This could be challenging if you have teenagers whose calorie needs are quite high and may require a more substantial snack in between meals. However, with younger children, such as preschoolers or early elementary age kids, it could be an excellent way to foster healthy eating habits from a very early age. It may also be a useful strategy if your child (of any age) is overweight.

Farmer's Markets

One final suggestion to support "5-A-Day" is to join a CSA (Community Supported Agriculture) or go to a local Farmer's Market weekly.

Farmer's Markets are a great way for you and your kids to actively choose produce to buy for the week. Seasonal, freshly picked fruits and vegetables are more flavorful, which encourages your child to like them and eat them. The Farmer's Market is also a fun, inviting place for your child to try new foods. When they see other kids their age walking around biting into a strawberry or apple, they too want to try it.

If you're not familiar with CSA's, they're a popular way for people to buy local, seasonal produce from a nearby farmer. There are many different arrangements, but usually you can choose how often your box is delivered or picked up, ranging from once/week to once/month. It can be a fun "present" that arrives with a variety of produce, depending on what's in season.

With both CSA and Farmer's Markets, you are not only buying fresh, ripe, nutrient-rich produce, but also providing a fun way to encourage your child to try new fruits and vegetables. In addition, you're showing your commitment to providing healthy food to you and your family.

To learn more about CSA's or to find a CSA farm near you, check out one of the following websites:

- www.localharvest.org/csa
- www.newfarm.org/farmlocator/index.php
- www.eatwellguide.org

STRATEGY # 3 :
"IT'S ALL ABOUT CHOICES"

This strategy is really useful for creating a "Win-Win" situation for you and your child. Your "Win" is that your child is eating fruits and vegetables. Your child's "Win" is that he or she has some control.

What I mean by control is that when a child is given a choice, she is part of the decision-making process and is less likely to refuse the fruits and vegetables. Both kids and adults want to have some control over our food choices, rather than being told what to eat.

Registered Dietitians frequently suggested offering choices as a way to get their kids to eat fruits and vegetables. There are many ways to go about offering choices. One approach is to give your child two vegetable options and allow him to choose which one he wants. For example, you might say, "Do you want green beans or carrots at dinner?" You might be wondering, "What if my child says he doesn't want green beans or carrots?" In this case, it becomes your job to choose what to serve. I recommend a simple response such as, "Ok, I'll decide which one you will have." Usually with time your child realizes he would rather make the decision himself.

Another approach frequently stated by Nutrition Experts was "It isn't a choice of *if* we are having a vegetable, but *which* vegetable to have". The idea here is that your child doesn't have a choice about having or not having a vegetable, but *does* have a choice about which one she eats.

I recommend offering no more than two vegetable options. That way your child isn't overwhelmed by too many choices and you don't become a short-order cook.

Another way Nutrition Experts said they provide choices is by asking their children for input on the grocery list.

By asking children what fruits and vegetables they want, you are engaging them in the process and helping them "take ownership" of their choices. The end result is that they're less likely to complain and more likely to really eat the fruits and vegetables.

If your child is too young to verbalize his choices, then another way to get input is to take him along to the grocery store or Farmer's Market where he can see the fruits and vegetables to pick out his choices. The combination of asking for input and having your child help with the shopping directly involves them in the process of making healthy choices.

Many Registered Dietitians suggested planting your own garden.

This is a great opportunity to involve your kids in the whole process from choosing what to plant, watching it grow, helping to harvest and then enjoying the fruits of their labor. If your children are old enough, you can ask them to pick from the garden the items you will need for preparing the meal. The older children can also wash, cut up and prepare that portion of the meal. If your child is preschool age, choose jobs that are age-appropriate and safe.

Speaking Of Preschoolers . . .

A fun concept to introduce to your child is **"Eat a Rainbow"**, which can be separate or in conjunction with planting a garden. The idea is to choose fruits and vegetables throughout the day that resemble the colors of a rainbow. By doing so, it can make choosing and eating fruits and vegetables more fun, and your child will eat a greater variety of vitamins and minerals.

STRATEGY # 4 : "IT'S WHAT WE DO"

A common response from Nutrition Experts involved a*utomatically* serving fruits and vegetables .

I mentioned this earlier and want to explain how it works. They frequently stated, "I *always* serve them. My kids are used to it." In other words, it's "the norm" or the standard in these households for fruits and vegetables to be served at meals and snacks. **It's what these kids expect to be served.**

Combined with that, the parent/dietitian *expects* the child to eat them. When it comes to meals, fruits and vegetables are a common part of what they eat regularly.

Another comment related to Strategy #4 was "There's no big deal. It's always served as part of a standard dinner meal". In an ideal world, starting this approach when your child is a toddler works to your advantage because it becomes "all they know" or the standard expectation to eat fruits and vegetables several times each day. However, even if your kids are older, new patterns and expectations can be established. It will take persistence on your part, but it *is* doable.

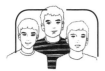

I believe this strategy has been a key to the success I've had with getting my boys to eat fruits and vegetables.

No Substitutes . . .

Another example of the "It's What We Do" strategy is the **No Substitutes Rule**. The principle is to allow your child to eat as little or as much as he wants from what is served on the plate; however, there will be no alternatives served until the next meal. This was expressed as, "That's what's for dinner".

One of the benefits of using this approach is that you avoid becoming a Short-Order Cook. By teaching your child that her option is what is served, she will eat it if she's hungry enough or wait until the next meal. The reality is, your child won't be harmed or "starve" by skipping a meal and they learn that negotiating to get "something else to eat" isn't an option.

Some parents feel this approach is too rigid.

A variation that may be more comfortable for you is to have **one standard alternative**. A few key components to making this approach work are the following:
1. The alternative is for the fruit and vegetable only (not the whole meal)
2. The alternative is always the same
3. The alternative is not overly desirable

For example, if your child says, "I don't want salad", then your matter-of-fact response is, "The only other choice is baby carrots. Which do you want?" Several weeks (or sometimes months) of baby carrots is likely to get tiresome, which might encourage your child to try some other choices. But even if he doesn't burn out on carrots every day, it's better than a battle at the table or no vegetable at all.

Another principle of "It's What We Do" is the parents eating the same foods the child is served.

Sometimes referred to as **Modeling**, this approach of leading by example, can be very effective *over time* in getting your child to eat vegetables with little or no complaining. Instead of using the "because I said so" approach, showing the importance of eating healthy food by doing so yourself is much more convincing, especially with younger children. Then by the time they are teenagers, they're usually convinced, even if they won't admit it.

37 Ideas to Get More Vegetables. . .

1. Add vegetables to pasta sauce

2. Add vegetables to soup, stew or casserole

3. Add fruit to oatmeal or cereal

4. Mix fruit in smoothies (see recipe on *page 164*)

5. Add fruit to yogurt

6. Serve vegetables with dip (See dip ideas on *page 141*)

7. Serve vegetables right before dinner

8. Serve vegetables while doing homework

9. Have cut up vegetables available on the table

10. Have cut up fruit available in the fridge

11. Always have fruit in a bowl on the counter

12. Serve vegetables as a snack in the car when going to activities

13. Only snacks between meals are fruits and vegetables

14. Serve a fruit or vegetable before any other snack

15. Eat fruits and vegetables yourself

16. Fruit is dessert every other day

17. Offer lots of variety

18. Prepare vegetables a variety of ways : raw, steamed, stir-fry, grilled.

19. Offer 1 alternative if vegetable or fruit served is rejected.

20. Offer 2 vegetable options and let your child choose

21. Offer fruits and vegetables frequently

22. Serve 2 vegetables at dinner

23. Serve a larger portion of favorite fruits and vegetables; Smaller portion when serving unpopular fruit or vegetable

24. Serve a larger portion of fruit and smaller portion of vegetable, but both are on the plate

25. No dessert if vegetable is not eaten or tried

26. Sprinkle vegetables with Parmesan cheese

27. Serve vegetables with low fat cheese sauce (see recipe on *page 142*)

28. Cook Sweet Potato Fries (see *page 140*)

29. Use seasonings on vegetables: garlic or garlic powder, lemon, chili powder, Mrs. Dash

30. Let your child choose his or her fruit for each meal

31. Ask your child to help wash fruits and vegetables for dinner

32. Ask your child to help cut up the fruit and vegetable for dinner

33. Each child chooses a fruit and vegetable at the grocery store

34. Shop together for fruits and vegetables at the Farmer's Market

35. Try "one bite"

36. Re-try the rejected vegetable about once/month

37. Let your child choose 2 vegetables to plant in the garden

Great Tips!

Sweet Potato Fries

Ingredients:
Look for one of these brands of sweet potato fries
in the freezer section of your grocery store or go
to the website and click on "store locator" to
find which store in your area stocks them:

Alexia Sweet Potato Julienne Fries:
www.alexiafoods.com, (866) 484-8676.

McCain Crinkle Cut Sweet Potato Fries:
www.mccainpotatoes.com, (877) 804-6198.

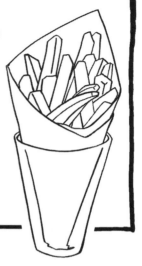

Preparation:
1. Place on a baking sheet and bake according to package directions.
2. Serve.

Note: My kids like cinnamon and/or black pepper sprinkled on the fries before baking to create a sweet, savory flavor.

Although the frozen versions are a little higher in calories and fat, they are equivalent in fiber and vitamin A compared to a homemade version. Better yet, they are *much healthier* **than restaurant French fries** and very convenient! So give them a try.

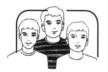

Many kids really like the taste of sweet potato fries because they're slightly sweet, yet have some of the same characteristics of traditional French fries. Although homemade sweet potato fries are the healthiest option, I have to admit, my boys like the frozen ones a whole lot better than my homemade recipe. Be sure to choose brands with **no more than 5 grams Total Fat / Serving.**

What's for Dipping

One great way to encourage your child to eat more vegetables is to provide a dip that adds flavor and ideally nutrition. But even if the dip doesn't provide nutrition, the vegetables will and, therefore, it's worth serving.

Here are several options to try:

- Salsa   · BBQ Sauce   · Hummus   · Ketchup
- Mustard   · Yogurt   · Peanut Butter
- Homemade Cheese Sauce (see recipe next page)
- Salad Dressing : *I recommend "light" or low fat salad dressings* — Ranch, Italian, Raspberry Vinaigrette, Soy Sesame Vinaigrette

Yummy Ranch Dip

Ingredients:
2 (6oz.) containers nonfat, plain yogurt
1 (1 oz.) package dry Original Ranch dressing mix

In a medium bowl, whisk together yogurt and dressing mix until well blended.
Refrigerate at least 1 hour.
Makes 1 ½ cups.

Serve with carrot sticks, celery sticks, cucumber slices, or sweet bell pepper strips.

Nutrition per serving (2 Tablespoons):

22 Calories, 0g Total Fat, 0g Saturated Fat, 1mg Cholesterol, 190mg Sodium, 3.5g Carbohydrate, 0g Fiber, 1g Protein

NOTE: If desired, add about ¼ cup nonfat or 1% milk to above ingredients. Whisk together and refrigerate to use as salad dressing.

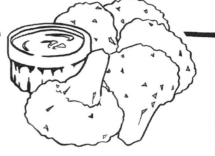

Kid-Friendly Cheese Sauce

Ingredients:
2 tablespoons Wondra flour
1 cup nonfat milk
½ cup (2 oz.) shredded sharp cheddar cheese
¼ teaspoon salt
Spices as desired*

Preparation:
1. Combine Wondra flour and nonfat milk in a small, heavy saucepan.
2. Cook over medium-high heat and stir regularly until bubbles rise (do not bring to a full boil).
3. Reduce heat to medium and cook until thickened, stirring occasionally.
4. Remove from heat; add cheese, salt and any additional spices.
5. Cover and let stand for about 3 minutes, until cheese is melted.
6. Stir and serve.
Makes 1-¼ Cups

add spices, such as black pepper, chili powder, cayenne pepper or other favorites

Nutrition per serving (2 Tablespoons):

45 Calories, 2g Total Fat, 1.5g Saturated Fat, 8mg Cholesterol, 129mg Sodium, 3g Carbohydrate, 0g Fiber, 3g Protein

NOTE: This sauce works well for macaroni and cheese too! You may need to double the recipe, depending on how much macaroni you are cooking.

The Bottom Line :

Your job as a parent is to encourage your child to make healthy choices (including at least five servings of fruits and vegetables daily), while maintaining a peaceful, low stress environment at meal and snack times. By choosing strategies that work for other Moms and their kids, you're more likely to achieve this goal.

Your Game Plan :

You might want to review the Daily Action Steps on *page 42* or review the 4 Strategies below to help you create your Game Plan.

Strategy #1 : The Bite Rule
Strategy #2 : 5-A-Day Everyday
Strategy #3 : It's All About Choices
Strategy #4 : It's What We Do

What do you want to do differently to help your child eat more fruits and vegetables?

1. _____

2. _____

3. _____

Share Your Thoughts . . .

I'd love to hear what Daily Action Steps you've tried or what you're doing differently that's working.   Have you tried any of the Strategies? Please tell me about your results…any benefits or challenges you've had. Are there any great tips or ideas you'd like to share?

**Please go to my website: www.400moms.com
or send me an e-mail at Jill@400moms.com
to share your thoughts and comments!**

CHAPTER 8

WHAT'S FOR DESSERT?

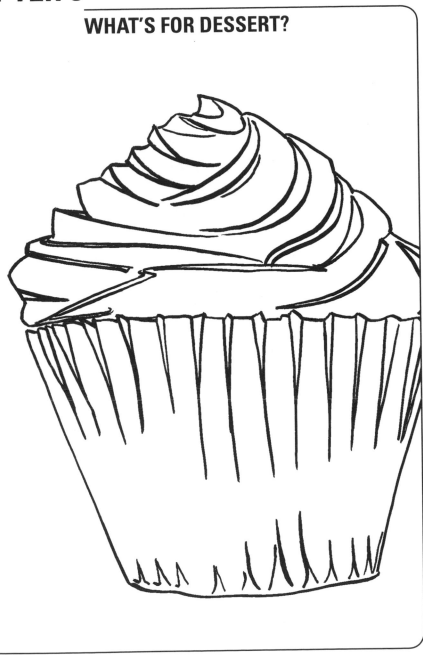

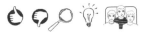

"What's for Dessert?"

I love them. My husband loves them.
And guess what….. my kids love them too.
I don't know if there's a genetic component to loving sweets,
but if there is, my kids got a double dose.

That being said, we eat sweets in moderation, choose the healthier options and enjoy them when we have them. My hope is that you'll be able to do the same after reading this chapter.

Moms frequently ask me "How much is too much?" when it comes to sweets. It's a challenging question that doesn't have a straight-forward or consensus answer, but I'll give my opinions and recommendations throughout this chapter. Keep in mind that if anyone in your family is more sensitive to sugar or has a medical condition that is affected by sugar intake, you should consult your physician or Registered Dietitian for individualized recommendations.

Just like soda and fast food, our consumption of sweets (desserts and candy) has increased significantly over the last 25 years.

Based on a USDA Nutrition Survey, the average American consumed **88 grams of added sugar daily!** That's the same as pouring 22 packets of sugar into your mouth.

The American Heart Association recommends women decrease sugar consumption to no more than 100 calories per day (this is equal to about 24 grams of added sugar), and men decrease sugar intake to no more than 150 calories (about 36 grams of added sugar per day).

Although the American Heart Association has not made a specific recommendation for kids, I recommend no more than 6 teaspoons of added sugar per day because preschool and elementary-aged kids need about the same number of calories as women, so the amount of sugar consumed should be similar.

The USDA is a little more liberal with its sugar guidelines, recommending no more than 40 grams per day for all Americans.

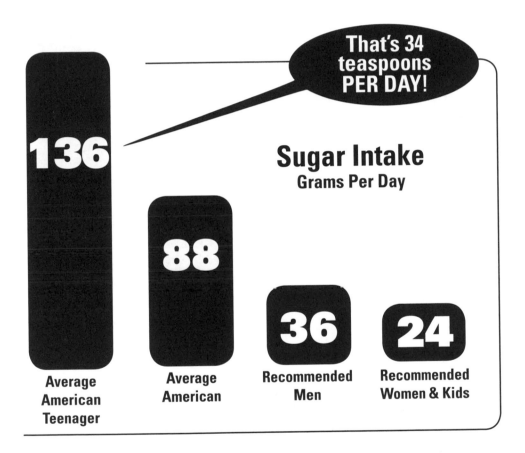

It's important to clarify that the sugar recommendations do not include naturally- occurring sugar found in milk, vegetables and fruit, but only the sugar that gets added to foods, such as condiments, snacks, yogurt, soda and desserts.

Check food labels to get an idea of how much added sugar you and your child currently eat.

THE GOAL IS :

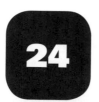

No more than 24 grams of added per day for women and kids. *(That's 6 teaspoons)* *Teenagers in America average 136 grams.* *(That's 34 teaspoons)*

No more than 36 grams of added sugar per day for men. *(That's 9 teaspoons)* *Americans average 88 grams.* *(That's 22 teaspoons)*

I know it isn't fair that men get more sugar, but the recommendation is based on how many daily calories your body needs. Men need about 2200 calories per day. Women need about 1800 calories per day.

Let's take a look at some examples:

1 cup of Kellogg's Fruit Loops cereal has 12 grams of sugar…already halfway to the recommended daily maximum for a child.

Add 3 Nabisco Oreos at lunch, which have 14 grams of sugar….your child is over the recommended 24 grams of sugar per day.

Grams Of Sugar In . . .

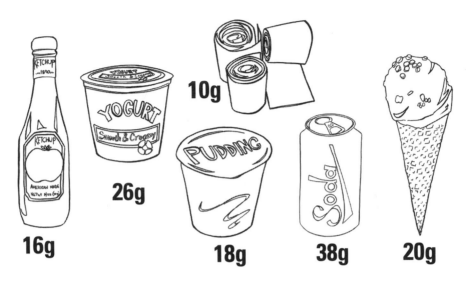

10g

26g

16g   **18g**   **38g**   **20g**

Here are just a few more examples :

¼ cup ketchup = 16 grams of sugar

6 oz. Yoplait Strawberry yogurt = 26 grams of sugar

½ cup Jello pudding = 18 grams of sugar

Betty Crocker Fruit by the Foot = 10 grams of sugar

One Nestle Vanilla Drumstick ice cream cone = 20 grams of sugar

A 12 oz. can of regular soda has **38-52 grams of sugar** depending on which flavor and brand you choose. Yes, that equals 1 to 2 days' worth of sugar, depending on whether you are a man, woman or child! **And that was for 12 oz., not the average 20oz. bottle of soda that most people drink today.**

Reading the labels, however, can get tricky because many foods have naturally occurring sugar *and* added sugar. For example, cereals with dried fruit, yogurt, pudding and trail mix have both types of sugar. Unfortunately, the current Nutrition Facts label doesn't differentiate each type of sugar, so there's no easy way to determine how much is naturally-occurring sugar and how much is added sugar in a particular food.

Why is Sugar a Problem?

Besides causing cavities, you might be wondering, "What exactly is the problem with high sugar intake?" Research is on-going to determine if there's a direct link between sugar intake and specific chronic diseases, but we do know that high-sugar foods push out more healthful choices and add extra calories.

As a parent, I know your job is to help your child *avoid* these health problems and lowering the amount of sugar your child eats can make a big difference!

High Sugar Diets =

HIGH Calories
LOW Fruits & Vegetables
LOW Vitamins & Minerals

According to USDA data, people who eat diets high in sugar eat less fruits and vegetables and get less calcium, fiber, folate, vitamin A, vitamin C, vitamin E, zinc, magnesium and iron. So it's very likely that high sugar intake at least *contributes* to obesity, osteoporosis, diabetes, cancer and heart disease if not directly causing these conditions.

Keeping a Healthy Perspective

Although desserts and sweets offer little nutritional value, there's no evidence showing that enjoying occasional sweets is a health problem. As a matter of fact, I believe limiting dessert too much is not healthy either. **The key is keeping desserts to an "occasional" choice.** Your job as a parent is to teach your child healthy eating habits, not restrictive eating habits. If any food is completely denied (except for medical reasons, such as food allergies), it often becomes more desirable and has the potential to create food and eating issues later in life. So it's very important to establish a healthy balance, eating mostly healthy foods and enjoying occasional desserts, without creating family stress and food battles.

The Good, the Bad, and the Ugly

On the next few pages I've created lists of store-bought cookies and frozen desserts and how they measure up. The criteria I used to assess the "Worst" and "Best" choices are based on the amount of calories first, then saturated fat, total fat and sugar in that order. I didn't include Trans-Fat in my criteria because most companies have eliminated it from the ingredients, yet many of the products still have plenty of heart-clogging saturated fat.

For example, if two different cookies had the same high calories, then I looked at which one had more saturated fat and that cookie ranked "worse". If they had the same calories and saturated fat, then I compared the total fat and lastly, the sugar content.

On the Worst List, the desserts are "ranked" worst at the top of the list and less bad (but still unhealthy) at the bottom of the list. For the Best List, all choices are acceptable with the "Best of the Best" at the top of the list.

Be sure to notice the serving sizes listed in the tables. The standard for the Nutrition Facts label is about 30 grams per serving for cookies, so the number of cookies will vary depending on how much each cookie weighs. For ice cream, frozen yogurt and sorbet, the standard serving size is ½-cup. The weight of the ½ cup will vary, but the portion is the same. For example, ½-cup of Haagen Daz ice cream is 100- 110 grams, while ½ cup of Dreyer's Light ice cream is 60 grams. For ice cream bars and sandwiches the serving size is extremely variable, so check the package carefully.

It's also important to note that these lists are not all inclusive. Companies can change the ingredients in their products and frequently distribute different brands and varieties to different regions of the country. However, you can use my recommended criteria (on *page 158*) and compare your local brands to determine if what you buy falls into The Worst or The Best lists. Secondly, I didn't include every ice cream flavor or novelty on the WORST list. For example, there are several Ben & Jerry's ice cream flavors that contain 8 grams of saturated fat, which would qualify for the WORST list, but do not appear. Instead, I chose to provide a sampling of the unhealthiest choices.

Jill's Worst Picks :
Store-Bought Cookies

Brand & Type	Serving Size	Calories	Saturated Fat (grams)	TOTAL Fat (grams)	Sugar (grams)
Mother's Taffy Creme	2 (38g)	180	4	8	16
Mother's Vanilla Creme	2 (38g)	180	3	7	11
Pepperidge Farm Tahiti	2 (30g)	170	6	10	8
Pepperidge Farm Milano	3 (34g)	170	5	9	13
Nabisco Nutter Butter Crème Patties	5 (32g)	170	2.5	9	8
Keebler Peanut Butter Fudge Sticks	3 (29g)	160	5	9	12
Nabisco Chips Ahoy Reeses	2 (30g)	160	4.5	9	9
Pepperidge Farm Geneva	3 (31g)	160	4	9	8
Keebler Chips Deluxe Original	2 (30g)	160	3.5	8	9
Mother's Chocolate Chip	2 (32g)	160	3	8	11
Pepperidge Farm Lemon	4 (32g)	160	3	8	8
Nabisco Chips Ahoy	3 (33g)	160	2.5	8	11
Keebler Fudge Sticks	3 (29g)	150	5	8	15
Keebler Fudge Stripes	3 (31g)	150	4.5	7	10
Nabisco Chips Ahoy Heath	2 (30g)	150	4	8	9
Pepperidge Farm Brussels	3 (30g)	150	4	7	11
Nabisco Oreo Chocolate	2 (30g)	150	2.5	7	13
Keebler Coconut Dreams	2 (28g)	140	6	8	10
Keebler Fudge Shoppe Grasshopper	4 (29g)	140	5	7	12
Keebler Deluxe Grahams	3 (27g)	140	4.5	7	10
Pepperidge Farm Dbl. Chocolate Milano	2 (27g)	140	4	8	10
Pepperidge Farm Dbl Chocolate Nantucket	1 (26g)	140	3	7	8
Pepperidge Farm Soft Baked Sausalito	1 (31g)	140	3	6	10
Pepperidge Farm Soft Baked Nantucket	1 (31g)	140	3	6	10
Pepperidge Farm Soft Baked Montauk	1 (31g)	140	3	6	10
Pepperidge Farm Soft Baked Captiva	1 (31g)	140	3	6	10
Nabisco Oreo Mint	2 (29g)	140	2.5	7	13
Keebler Chips Deluxe Soft 'n Chewy	2 (33g)	140	2.5	6	9
Pepperidge Farm Verona	3 (32g)	140	2.5	5	9
Pepperidge Farm Milano Melts	2 (27g)	140	2	7	11
Pepperidge Farm Mint Milano	2 (25g)	130	5	7	8
Pepperidge Farm Orange Milano	2 (25g)	130	5	7	8
Pepperidge Farm Raspberry Milano	2 (25g)	130	4.5	7	8
Pepperidge Farm Sausalito	1 (26g)	130	3.5	6	10
Pepperidge Farm Tahoe	1 (26g)	130	3.5	6	10
Pepperidge Farm Chesapeake	1 (26g)	130	3.5	6	10
Pepperidge Farm Bordeaux	4 (27g)	130	3.5	5	12
Pepperidge Farm Nantucket	1 (26g)	130	3	6	8
Pepperidge Farm Montauk	1 (26g)	130	3	6	7
Pepperidge Farm Chessman	3 (26g)	120	3	5	5

Jill's BEST Picks :
Store-Bought Cookies

Brand & Type	Serving Size	Calories	Saturated Fat (grams)	TOTAL Fat (grams)	Sugar (grams)
Nabisco Fat-Free Fig Newtons	2 (29g)	90	0	0	12
Snackwell's Devil's Food	2 (32g)	100	0	0	14
Nabisco Raspberry Newtons	2 (29g)	100	0	1.5	13
Nabisco Strawberry Newtons	2 (29g)	100	0	1.5	13
Nabisco 100-cal Oreo Thin Crisps	1pkg. (23g)	100	0	2	8
Nabisco 100-cal Chips Ahoy	1pkg. (23g)	100	0.5	3	7
Keebler Right Bites Cocolate Chip	1pouch (21g)	100	1	3	8
Nabisco 100-cal Lorna Doone	1pkg. (21g)	100	1.5	3	6
Keebler Right Bites Mini Brownies	1 pouch (21g)*	100	1.5	4	7
Nabisco Fig Newtons (regular)	2 (31g)	110	0	2	12
Snackwell's Crème Sandwich	2 (25g)	110	1	3	9
Nabisco Reduced Fat Nilla Wafers	8 (29g)	120	0	2	12
Nabisco Ginger Snaps	4 (28g)	120	0	2.5	11
Nabisco Cinnamon lowfat Graham Crackers	8 (31g)	120	0	2	8
Kashi Oatmeal Raisin Flax	1 (30g)	130	0	4.5	7
Nabisco Honey Graham Crackers	8 (31g)	130	0.5	3	8
Nabisco Teddy Grahams	24 (30g)	130	0.5	4	8
Nabisco Chocolate Graham Crackers	8 (30g)	130	1	3	8
Pepperidge Farm Gingerman	4 (28g)	130	1.5	3.5	13
Pepperidge Farm Soft Baked Santa Cruz	1 (31g)	130	1.5	4.5	13
Mother's Oatmeal	2 (27g)	130	1.5	5	8
Kashi Oatmeal Dark Chocolate	1 (30g)	130	1.5	5	8
Trader Joe's Cinnamon Schoolbook	15 (30g)	130	2	4	8
Nabisco Animal Crackers	17 (31g)	140	0.5	4	8
Nabisco Vanilla Wafers (regular)	8 (30g)	140	1.5	6	11
Pepperidge Farm Soft Baked Sanibel	1pkg. (21g)	140	2	5	9

serving size is less than the standard of 30 grams.

NOTE: I did not include granola bars or cereal bars in these lists. However, many of them have similar nutritional content. I believe they should be considered a dessert, rather than a snack, because of the high sugar content.

Jill's Worst Picks :
Frozen Desserts
Ice Cream Bars, Cones & Sandwiches

Brand & Type	Serving Size	Calories	Saturated Fat (grams)	TOTAL Fat (grams)	Sugar (grams)
Good Humor					
Triple Chocolate Brownie Giant King	1 cone	380	10	14	38
Good Humor Chocolate Giant King	1 cone	360	9	17	32
It's It Original Ice Cream Sandwich	1 each	340	10	18	17
Nestle Vanilla Carmel Drumstick	1 each	310	9	16	24
Nestle Vanilla Fudge Drumstick	1 each	310	9	16	24
Nestle Chocolate Drumstick	1 each	300	9	17	23
Nestle Vanilla Drumstick	1 each	290	9	16	20
Reeses Ice Cream Cup	1 bar	280	10	19	18
Good Humor Chocolate Chip Sandwich	1 each	270	6	10	25
Klondike Bar Reeses	1 bar	260	11	16	20
Klondike Bar Original Vanilla	1 bar	250	11	14	23
Good Humor King Cone	1 cone	240	7	12	20
Good Humor Sundae Cone	1 cone	240	7	12	18
Good Humor Oreo Bar	1 bar	240	6	13	19
Klondike Bar Heath	1 bar	230	11	15	20
Good Humor Strawberry Shortcake	1 bar	230	3.5	10	17
Good Humor Giant Neapolitan Sandwich	1 each	220	3	5	22
Good Humor Giant Vanilla Sandwich	1 each	220	3	5	21
Good Humor Snack Pops	2 bars	210	10	13	18
Good Humor Chocolate Éclair	1 bar	210	4	9	16
Good Humor Toasted Almond	1 bar	210	3.5	10	15
Weight Watchers English Toffee Crunch	2 bars	200	9	12	20
Mounds Bar	1 bar	190	9	11	18
Good Humor Dark or Milk Chocolate	1 bar	180	9	13	12
Klondike Bar Ice Cream Sandwich	1 each	180	2.5	4.5	16
York Ice Cream	1 bar	170	7	10	15
Weight Watchers Ice Cream Candy Bar	1 bar	140	3.5	9	11
Good Humor Cookies & Cream	1 bar	90	1	1.5	10

Jill's Worst Picks :
Frozen Desserts
Ice Cream Bars, Frozen Yogurt & Sorbet

Brand & Type	Serving Size	Calories	Saturated Fat (grams)	TOTAL Fat (grams)	Sugar (grams)
Ice Cream					
Ben & Jerry's Peanut Butter Cup	½ cup	350	13	24	25
Haagen-Dazs Chocolate Peanut Butter	½ cup	340	10	23	22
Ben & Jerry's NY Super Fudge Chunk	½ cup	300	11	20	25
Haagen-Dazs Chocolate Chocolate Chip	½ cup	300	11	19	22
Haagen-Dazs Vanilla Swiss Almond	½ cup	300	10	20	21
Ben & Jerry's Everything But The...	½ cup	300	11	17	28
Haagen-Dazs Java Chip	½ cup	290	11	17	28
Haagen-Dazs Pistachio	½ cup	290	10	20	16
Ben & Jerry's Chunky Monkey	½ cup	290	9	17	28
Ben & Jerry's Cinnamon Buns	½ cup	290	9	15	28
Haagen-Dazs Rocky Road	½ cup	290	8	17	22
Ben & Jerry's S'mores	½ cup	290	8	15	27
Ben & Jerry's Vanilla Heath Bar	½ cup	280	10	17	27
Ben & Jerry's Coffee Heath Bar Crunch	½ cup	280	10	16	27
Ben & Jerry's Phish Food	½ cup	280	8	13	27
Ben & Jerry's American Dream	½ cup	280	10	15	25
Ben & Jerry's Imagine Whirled Peace	½ cup	270	11	16	23
Haagen-Dazs Rum Raisin	½ cup	260	10	17	20
Haagen-Dazs Chocolate	½ cup	260	10	17	19
Ben & Jerry's Cake Batter	½ cup	260	9	14	24
Haagen-Dazs Vanilla	½ cup	250	10	17	19
Haagen-Dazs Strawberry	½ cup	250	9	16	20
Ben & Jerry's Cherry Garcia	½ cup	240	9	13	23
Haagen-Dazs Pineapple Coconut	½ cup	230	8	13	23
Ben & Jerry's Mint Chocolate Cookie	½ cup	220	7	13	17
Frozen Yogurt					
Ben & Jerry's Phish Food	½ cup	240	4.5	6	27
Ben & Jerry's Greek Banana Peanut Butter	½ cup	210	2.5	8	26
Ben & Jerry's Cherry Garcia	½ cup	200	2	3	27
Ben & Jerry's Half Baked	½ cup	200	1.5	3	24
Ben & Jerry's Greek Blueberry Vanilla	½ cup	200	3	7	23
Ben & Jerry's Greek Raspberry Fudge Chunk	½ cup	200	5	7	25
Ben & Jerry's Chocolate Fudge Brownie	½ cup	180	1.5	2.5	25
Ben & Jerry's Greek Strawberry Shortcake	½ cup	180	3	5	21
Haagen-Dazs Vanilla	½ cup	170	1	2.5	21

Jill's BEST Picks :
Frozen Desserts
Ice Cream Bars, Cones & Sandwiches

Brand & Type	Serving Size	Calories	Saturated Fat (grams)	TOTAL Fat (grams)	Sugar (grams)
Dreyer's Fruit Bar no added sugar*	1 bar	25	0	0	2*
Breyer's Pure Fruit Bar	1 bar	40	0	0	9
Fudgesicle Fat Free Bar	1 bar	60	0	0	11
Dreyer's All Natural Fruit Bar	1 bar	80	0	0	20
Fudgesicle no added sugar*	2 pops	80	1	1.5	5*
Weight Watchers Giant Latte Bar	1 bar	90	0.5	1	15
Good Humor Cookies & Cream	1 bar	90	1	1.5	10
Skinny Cow Fudge Bar	1 bar	100	0.5	1	13
Weight Watchers Giant Chocolate Fudge Bar	1 bar	100	0.5	1	15
Cremesicle (Orange or Raspberry)	1 bar	100	1	2	12
Fudgesicle Original	1 bar	100	1	2	14
Skinny Cow Mini Fudge Pops	2 bars	100	1	2	14
Skinny Cow Chocolate Truffle Bar	1 bar	100	2	2.5	11
Skinny Cow Cookies 'n Cream Truffle Bar	1 bar	100	2	3	12
Skinny Cow Caramel Truffle Bar	1 bar	100	2.5	1.5	11
Skinny Cow Mint Truffle Bar	1 bar	100	2.5	1.5	11
Good Humor Vanilla Sandwich	1 each	140	1.5	3	13
Skinny Cow Vanilla Ice Cream Sandwich	1 each	150	1	2	15
Skinny Cow Mint Ice Cream Sandwich	1 each	150	1	2	15
Skinny Cow Chocolate Peanut Butter Ice Cream Sandwich	1 each	150	1	2.5	15
Skinny Cow Cookies 'n Cream Ice Cream Sandwich	1 each	150	1	2	15
Skinny Cow Strawberry Shortcake Ice Cream Sandwich	1 each	150	1	2	15
Skinny Cow Chocolate w/ Fudge Cone	1 cone	150	2	3	15
Skinny Cow Mint w/ Fudge Cone	1 cone	150	2	3	17
Skinny Cow Vanilla w/ Caramel cone	1 cone	150	2	3	17

Contains artificial sweeteners and sugar alcohols not accounted for in chart

Jill's BEST Picks :
Frozen Desserts
Ice Cream, Frozen Yogurt & Sorbet

Brand & Type	Serving Size	Calories	Saturated Fat (grams)	TOTAL Fat (grams)	Sugar (grams)
Frozen Yogurt					
Dreyer's Yogurt Blends Vanilla Fat Free	½ cup	90	0	0	14
Dreyer's Yogurt Blends Peach	½ cup	100	1.5	2.5	14
Dreyer's Yogurt Blends Vanilla	½ cup	100	1.5	3	13
Dreyer's Yogurt Blends Chocolate Fudge Brownie	½ cup	120	2	3.5	14
Dreyer's Yogurt Blends Cookies 'n Cream	½ cup	120	2	3.5	15
Dreyer's Yogurt Blends Caramel Praline Crunch	½ cup	120	2	3.5	16
Ice Cream					
Dreyer's Slow Churned Light Neapolitan	½ cup	90	2	3	12
Dreyer's Slow Churned Light French Vanilla	½ cup	100	2	3.5	11
Dreyer's Slow Churned Light Vanilla Bean	½ cup	100	2	3.5	12
Dreyer's Slow Churned Light Chocolate	½ cup	100	2	3.5	13
Dreyer's Slow Churned Light Rocky Road	½ cup	110	1	2.5	14
Dreyer's Slow Churned Light Caramel Delight	½ cup	110	1.5	2	16
Dreyer's Slow Churned Light Cookies 'n Cream	½ cup	120	1.5	2.5	13
Skinny Cow Dulce de Leche	container	150	0.5	1	20
Skinny Cow Strawberry Shortcake	container	150	0.5	1	22
Skinny Cow Chocolate Fudge Brownie	container	150	1	2	17
Skinny Cow Cookies 'n Cream	container	150	1	2	17
Skinny Cow Caramel Cone	container	160	2	2.5	21
Sorbet					
Haagen-Dazs Lemon	½ cup	120	0	0	27
Haagen-Dazs Raspberry	½ cup	120	0	0	27
Haagen-Dazs Strawberry	½ cup	130	0	0	28
Haagen-Dazs Orchard Peach	½ cup	130	0	0	30
Haagen-Dazs Mango	½ cup	150	0	0	36

Dreyer's and Edy's Brand are made by the same company

Jill's Dessert Criteria

It's important to know that the WORST list includes Ben & Jerry's and Haagen Daz frozen yogurts. Although these products are "healthier" than the ice cream, they are too high in calories to make the BEST list. Also notice that sorbet is listed on the BEST list. Since it meets the calorie and fat criteria, I've included it, but I want to emphasize that sorbet provides a real whollop of sugar (6 to 9 teaspoons per ½ cup)!

Also be aware that the company Dreyer's, which is available on the West coast, also owns and produces the Edy's brand of ice cream available on the East Coast. The product should be the same, but check the labeling to confirm the nutrition information is the same.

Finally, I've included a few desserts that contain artificial sweeteners. If you don't want to provide these choices to your children, there are still many dessert choices that are low in fat.

Since the reality is most families are going to have desserts in the house, why not make those options as "healthy" as possible. I put healthy in quotations because desserts are considered "extras", with little or no nutritional value, so they can't really be called healthy. But since some are nutritionally better than others, I'm calling those the "healthy" choices.

Jill's Dessert Criteria :
150 calories or less
2 grams of saturated fat or less

When purchasing desserts for my children I check the calories first and provide serving sizes that are no more than 150 calories. That way the "empty calories" my kids are eating from dessert is kept to a minimum.

What's Worse…High Fat or High Sugar?

I don't know if you've noticed, but when a food manufacturer lowers or removes the fat in a product, the sugar content usually goes up. And if they take sugar out of a product, oftentimes the fat content goes up. Which leads to the question: "Which is worse . . . fat or sugar?"

Well, neither is good, but when we're talking about desserts, my opinion is that fat is worse, especially if it's saturated or trans-fat.

Too much fat leads to excessive calories, too much weight gain, high cholesterol and eventually heart disease and/or diabetes. To make matters worse, the high fat and high sugar are oftentimes in the same food, such as snacks and desserts.

The strategy that works best is:

Choose sweets with no more than 150 calories - AND - provide the serving size listed on the package

For example, the Nutrition Facts label lists 2 Nabisco Fig Newtons as a serving for 110 calories, whereas Nabisco Animal Crackers has a serving size of 17 crackers for 140 calories. Both of these cookies are an appropriate serving size and are within 150 calories. By using this strategy you will automatically limit how much fat and sugar is in your child's dessert.

Homemade vs. Store-Bought . . . Is There a Difference?

I know finding time to make desserts can be a challenge for many moms, but if you're inclined to make your own cookies, cakes, muffins or pies, then homemade desserts definitely have the potential to be healthier than store-bought goodies. Why? Because you have control over what ingredients go into the dessert. By making a few modifications in the amount of sugar, fat and/or type of flour you use, the desserts can become significantly healthier than a store-bought version.

Below are suggestions to improve the nutritional content of your homemade desserts.

Cut the sugar by 1/4 to 1/2.
Many recipes call for much more sugar than is needed to provide the right texture and make the dessert taste sweet. By decreasing the sugar gradually (i.e. starting with 1/4 less sugar than the recipe calls for) you can lower the calories and sugar while maintaining the desired texture. So if the cookie recipe calls for one cup of sugar, decrease to ¾ cup and keep all other ingredients the same.

Substitute half of the fat (butter, margarine or oil) with applesauce.
This works best with muffins, cakes and quick breads. The unsweetened applesauce maintains the necessary moisture, while significantly lowering the fat content. For example, if a recipe calls for ½ cup butter, I use ¼ cup butter + ¼ cup applesauce, which **cuts out 12-teaspoons of fat and 400 calories** with just one change!

Exchange 2 egg whites for 1 whole egg. This will reduce the unhealthy saturated fat and cholesterol in the dessert without changing the texture or flavor.

Replace half of the white flour with whole wheat flour. This will add fiber to your cookies, cakes, quick breads, muffins or pie crust. Many people like the nuttier flavor, so give it a try and see what you think!

Instead of a two-crust pie, make a fruit crisp with an oatmeal crumb topping. By eliminating two pie crusts and substituting the oatmeal topping, you significantly decrease the fat and calories compared to a fruit pie. Check out the Fruit Crisp recipe on *page 163*.

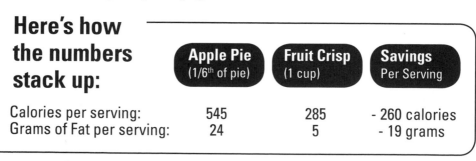

Here's how the numbers stack up:	Apple Pie (1/6th of pie)	Fruit Crisp (1 cup)	Savings Per Serving
Calories per serving:	545	285	- 260 calories
Grams of Fat per serving:	24	5	- 19 grams

Instead of regular ice cream, use low fat ice cream or light whipped cream as the topping on your pie or cake. This will cut the fat by *more than half* for the a la mode portion of your dessert.

Cranberry Crunch Bars

Ingredients:
2 tablespoons butter
4 cups mini marshmallows
2 cups crispy rice cereal
2 cups Honey Bunches of Oats cereal
1 cup quick-cooking oats
½ cup dried cranberries

Preparation:
1. Lightly grease a 9 X 13-inch baking dish.
2. In a large bowl, combine cereals, oats and cranberries.
3. In a medium pot, melt butter. Add marshmallows and stir frequently until completed melted.
4. Remove from heat; add cereal mixture to melted marshmallows.
5. Stir until marshmallow mixture is well distributed.
6. Spoon mixture into baking dish. Wet hands and spread cereal mixture evenly to edges of pan.
7. Let cool 1 hour before cutting into squares.
Makes 18 servings

Nutrition Information per serving :

122 calories, 2g Total Fat, 1g Saturated Fat, 3mg Cholesterol, 59mg Sodium, 26g Carbohydrate, 1g Fiber, 1g Protein

This is a mix between a chewy granola bar and a crispy rice cookie. You can substitute your favorite cereal or add 1/3 cup sliced almonds for variety.

Baked Apple Slices

Ingredients:
4 medium apples
1 tablespoon unbleached, all-purpose flour
2 tablespoons granulated sugar
1 teaspoon cinnamon
¼ teaspoon allspice
¼ cup water

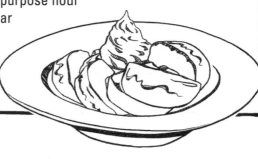

Preparation:
1. Preheat oven to 350°F.
2. Slice apples and place in a lightly greased, 9 X 13-inch baking dish.
3. In a small bowl combine flour, sugar, cinnamon and all spice with a wire whisk.
4. Sprinkle over apples and toss with your hands to coat evenly.
5. Drizzle water over the apples, cover with foil and bake for 40-45 minutes, or until apples are soft and easily pierced with a fork.

Makes 6 servings

Nutrition Information per serving:

86 calories, 0g Total Fat, 0g Saturated Fat, 0mg Cholesterol, 3mg Sodium, 23g Carbohydrate, 3g Fiber, 0g Protein

This makes a yummy dessert all by itself or you can add a dollop of light whipped cream to really make your kids happy. As a bonus, the dessert counts as a fruit serving!

Fantastic Fruit Crisp

Ingredients:
4 medium apples, peeled, cored and sliced
¾ cup dried cranberries (optional)
3 medium pears, peeled and chopped
2 tablespoons fresh orange juice
1 teaspoon orange zest
2 tablespoons unbleached white flour
2 tablespoons granulated sugar
1 teaspoon cinnamon
¼ cup water

Topping:
3/4 cup quick-cooking oats
3/4 cup unbleached, all-purpose flour
½ cup packed brown sugar
½ teaspoon baking powder
1 teaspoon cinnamon
¼ cup butter, melted

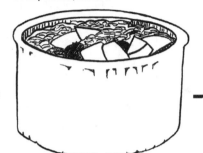

Preparation:
1. Preheat oven to 350°F.
2. In a large bowl, combine apples, cranberries, and pears; mix well.
3. In a small bowl combine flour, sugar, and cinnamon.
4. Sprinkle flour mixture over fruit and toss with your hands to coat evenly. Transfer to a 8 X 8-inch baking dish and stir in orange juice and orange zest.
5. Drizzle water over the fruit.
6. In a medium bowl, combine oats, flour, brown sugar, baking powder and cinnamon. Stir well.
7. Add melted butter and mix until crumbly mixture forms.
8. Pour over fruit and spread out evenly.
9. Bake at 350°F for 60-minutes, or until bubbling and topping is crisp.
Makes 9 servings

Nutrition Information per serving :

285 calories, 6g Total Fat, 3g Saturated Fat, 14mg Cholesterol, 98mg Sodium, 58g Carbohydrate, 6g Fiber, 2.5g Protein

This is a great dessert to make instead of pie because it eliminates the high fat, high calorie crust. Depending on the time of year, you can vary the fruit filling in this crisp to maximize the flavor using fruits in season. For example, you can substitute 1 cup fresh blueberries for the dried cranberries, or for a great summer fruit crisp try 6-8 medium nectarines, peaches or plums instead of the apples and pears.

Fruit Smoothie

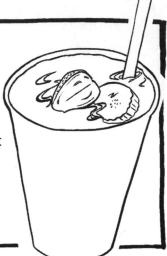

Ingredients :
1 ½ cups nonfat milk
2 (6 oz.) containers nonfat, fruit-flavored yogurt
3 medium frozen bananas, partially thawed
2 cups frozen strawberries

Preparation :
1. In a blender or food processor, add ingredients in the order listed.
2. Blend until smooth, adding more milk if needed to achieve desired consistency.
3. Pour into cups and serve.
   Makes 5 servings

Nutrition Information per serving :
167 calories, <1g Total Fat, 0g Saturated Fat, 2mg Cholesterol, 93mg Sodium, 35g Carbohydrate, 3g Fiber, 7g Protein.

Variation:
Substitute equivalent amount of fruits in season for bananas or strawberries and change yogurt flavor as desired.

NOTE :
This recipe makes several servings, so I pour the left-over into 8 oz. cups, cover with foil and store in the freezer. It makes a great dessert or after-school snack and can be quickly thawed by microwaving on HIGH for 30 seconds or so.

A great way to use up those overripe bananas! When our bananas get black spots, nobody will eat them, so I pop them in the freezer to use here. I like to use frozen or partially frozen fruit to make a thick smoothie. You can use fresh fruit, but the smoothie will be a thinner consistency.

The Bottom Line :

Teaching your child about moderation when it comes to unhealthy choices, including desserts, is part of healthy eating habits. By establishing how often and what types of sweets your family eats, you can help your child understand "moderation" and what a "healthy balance" means, without creating food fights.

Your Game Plan :

Three examples of strategies that could support your Game Plan are…

1. I will buy desserts from the "BEST Picks" list.
2. I will talk with my family about choosing 3 days of the week to be "dessert nights".
3. I will use Jill's dessert criteria (150-calories or less) when serving dessert.

Count how often and what kind of sweets and desserts your child eats currently. What will you change to ensure your child gets mostly nutritious foods without making dessert the "bad guy"?

1. _____

2. _____

3. _____

Share Your Thoughts . . .

Please tell me about your results… any benefits or challenges you've had? Are there any great tips or ideas you'd like to share?

**Please go to my website: www.400moms.com
or send me an e-mail at Jill@400moms.com
to share your thoughts and comments!**

CHAPTER 9

BEVERAGES

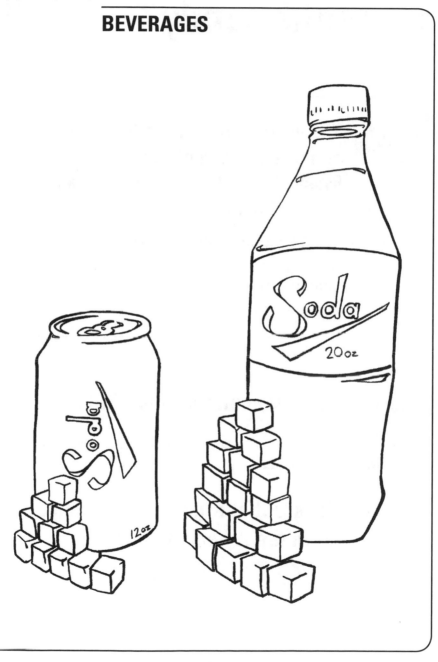

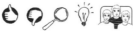

Beverages. . . or Liquid Candy?

The average American Teenager consumes ¾ cup of sugar EVERY DAY! Most–if not all–of that sugar has NO nutritional value.

Imagine a measuring cup ¾ full with sugar. Now picture your teenager taking that measuring cup, tilting his head back and pouring all that sugar into his mouth.

Where does all that sugar come from?

Mostly soda, but also other sweetened beverages, such as sports drinks, vitamin waters, juice or juice drinks, sweetened teas and coffee drinks.

These drinks are the largest single source of added sugar in the American diet.

Why Are Sodas & Sweet Drinks A Problem?

 Consuming sodas or sugar-sweetened beverages is associated with obesity in children and adolescents. As a matter of fact, the risk for obesity increases almost 60% with every additional soda a child drinks daily.

. . .

 Kids who consume a lot of sodas or sweetened beverages have a higher risk of heart disease as a child.

. . .

 Kids who drink soda are more likely to be lacking in Vitamins A, D, and B12, along with calcium and magnesium. All of which are important for building healthy bones, teeth and nervous system.

. . .

Adults who drink one or two sodas or sweetened beverages daily increase their risk of Type 2 Diabetes by 26%.

By drinking sweet drinks regularly, kids are more likely to become overweight or obese, which increases their risk of heart disease and diabetes now and as adults. I don't think that's what any parent wishes for his or her child.

DID YOU KNOW . . . From 1980 through 2012 obesity rates in U.S. kids have TRIPLED?

The most current data shows that 17% of children and adolescents (6-19 years old) are obese. When we combine the number of children who are overweight with the number of obese children, then the total is 32% – or 1 out of every 3 kids, is overweight or obese today!

Interestingly, the amount of sweetened beverages kids drink has increased over this same time frame. Food surveys show Americans' daily calories from soft drinks and sweet drinks have *quadrupled* between 1970 and 2010. These extra calories translate into extra weight gain for both kids and adults.

When we consume "liquid calories" we don't compensate by decreasing how much food we eat. In other words, the calories from sweetened beverages become "extra", or on top of what we normally eat, leading to higher daily calorie intake and ultimately, weight gain.

For example, one 12-ounce soda averages 150 calories. If your child drinks one soda every day while keeping food the same, he or she will gain *15 pounds in a year!* That's 15 pounds from liquid sugar.

Keep in mind that these sugar calories don't come from just soda, but from the many varieties of sweetened beverages kids drink daily.

To make matters worse, these sweet drinks are replacing the milk kids' bodies need! So instead of getting the calcium, vitamins and protein for bone and muscle growth, kids are getting sugar, caffeine, "empty calories" and a big dose of risk for future health problems. Not only is calcium important for building strong bones, but it's also important for keeping blood vessels healthy, regulating blood pressure, balancing hormones and helping the nervous system function properly. So it's really important that kids get the calcium their growing bodies need.

What Should Your Child Be Drinking?
Well, here's what Nutrition Experts let their kids drink:

 77% 77% of Registered Dietitians report their kids drink *2 or more* 8 oz. servings of Milk daily (includes cow's milk, enriched soy milk or enriched rice milk)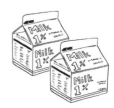

 87% 87% of Registered Dietitians report their kids drink *2 or more* 8 oz. servings of Water daily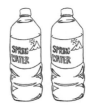

 54% 54% of Registered Dietitians rarely provide soda to their kids and **80%** allow soda *no more than once/week*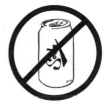

 62% 62% of Registered Dietitians provide *4 ounces* of juice every other day *or less*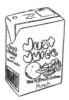

 73% 73% of Registered Dietitians provide "other sweetened beverages" *no more than once/week*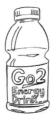

What I take from this data is that most Nutrition Experts regularly serve their children water and milk. Occasionally they serve juice (about every other day) and rarely do they allow soda and other sweetened beverages. In my survey, a frequent comment made by Nutrition Experts was "We only have soda on special occasions."

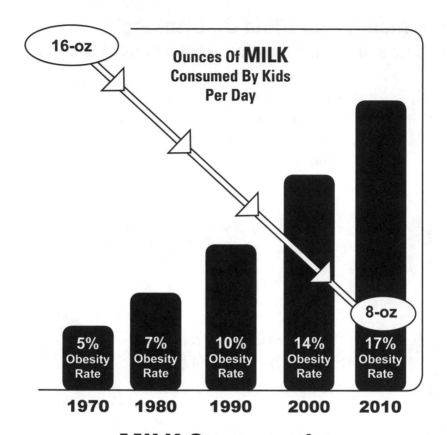

MILK Consumption
vs
Childhood Obesity Rates

This chart illustrates how the milk consumed by children has steadily DECLINED by 50% since 1970, while Childhood Obesity Rates have TRIPLED. Based on statistics from the USDA and other sources, children consumed 16 ounces of milk per day in 1970 and now drink about 8 ounces per day. And 2 out of 4 teens don't drink any milk at all.

Obesity Rates for children have climbed from 5% to 17% during this period. The Obesity Rate continues to climb as children become adults. The Obesity Rate for adults in the USA is now over 35%.

**77% of Nutrition Experts give their children
16 ounces of milk per day or more.**

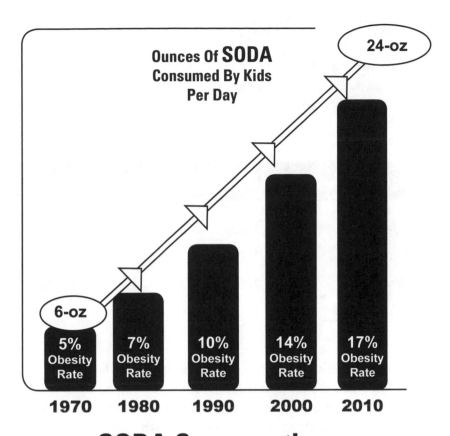

Ounces Of SODA
Consumed By Kids
Per Day

24-oz

6-oz

5% Obesity Rate	7% Obesity Rate	10% Obesity Rate	14% Obesity Rate	17% Obesity Rate
1970	1980	1990	2000	2010

SODA Consumption
vs
Childhood Obesity Rates

This chart goes a step further to show how soda consumption by children has QUADRUPLED since 1970 from 6 ounces of soda per day in 1970 to over 24 ounces per day by some estimates. This does not include the numerous other sweet drinks kids consume - energy drinks, sports drinks, juice drinks and sweet teas. So the reality is kids are drinking greater than 24 ounces of sweet drinks per day! It's clear to me that those Super-Sized Sodas and sweet drinks are a very significant contributor to weight gain in kids.

54% of Nutrition Experts RARELY give their
children soda and 80% allow soda
not more than once per week

How much milk does your child need?

How much water and milk your child needs depends on several factors, including age, activity and climate. In the chart below I've listed the number of cups of milk required each day to get the calcium your child needs based on his or her age.

Age	Calcium Needs (milligrams)	Milk/Day
1-3 years	700mg	2 1/3 cups
4-8 years	1000mg	3 1/3 cups
9-18 years	1,300 mg	4 1/3 cups

The amount of water your child needs depends somewhat on age, but mostly on your child's activity level and the weather. If your child is very active in sports or play, he will need more water than average. Offer water before, during and after physical activity to stay hydrated. In warm weather your child's fluid needs will also be greater because of increased fluid loss from sweating.

I recommend that you offer milk at least 3 times per day at mealtimes and then water in between meals. If your child is like many kids, she may not drink milk at school, so to ensure that she gets the recommended servings each day offer milk or another dairy product (such as low fat yogurt, string cheese or cottage cheese) at snack time and provide water in her lunch.

If your child really dislikes milk, this table provides some examples of foods containing calcium that can substitute for milk. I've included milk on the list to give you a way to compare the calcium content of other foods. These are averages of several brands, so the values may not match exactly with the brand you buy. Check the label for exact values. If you find your child is consistently below the recommended amount of calcium for his or her age, you should consider talking with your child's doctor or a Registered Dietitian to determine whether a calcium supplement would be advisable.

CALCIUM COMPARISONS

Product	Serving Size	Calcium (milligrams)	Calories	Sugar (grams)
Total cereal	¾ cup	1000	100	5
Total Raisin Bran	1 cup	1000	160	17
Total Corn Flakes	1 1/3 cups	1000	110	3
Nonfat Milk	**1 cup**	**300**	**90**	**12**
1% Milk	**1 cup**	**300**	**105**	**12**
Chocolate 1% Milk	1 cup	300	160	25
Soy milk (enriched)	1 cup	300	90-100	6-7
Rice milk (enriched)	1 cup	300	90-120	10-28
Almond milk (enriched)	1 cup	300	60-120	7-20
Basic 4 cereal	1 cup	250	200	13
Nonfat fruit yogurt	6 oz.	250	120	20
Fortified orange juice	1 cup	250	110	22
Cheese	1 oz.	200	100	0
Yoplait Light Yogurt*	6 ounces	200	100	14
Tofu	½ cup	150	40-70	0
Kix cereal	1 ¼ cups	150	110	3
Pudding	½ cup	150	90-100	17-19
Soybeans (green)	½ cup	130	125	0
Cottage Cheese	½ cup	100	80	3
Instant oatmeal	1 packet	100	130	12g
Yoplait Gogurt	1 tube	100	70	10g

Notice the difference in calories and sugar, depending on the product you choose. For example, a glass of milk has about the same calcium, but less calories and much less sugar than the fruit yogurt. That doesn't mean you shouldn't serve yogurt, but it's important to carefully choose the calcium sources you offer and limit the high sugar options.

If your child is overweight, you should consider serving "light" yogurts, which are sweetened with artificial sweeteners, so the sugar and calories are similar to milk.

Now back to beverages....

When packing a school lunch, many parents provide a "juice bag" or sports drink as the fluid when their child won't drink the milk at school.

I recommend you pack a small water bottle (ideally reusable) instead of juice to decrease the sugar calories, yet still provide the much needed fluid. You may get resistance from your child at first (change is not always easy), but I promise kids will drink the water when they're thirsty.

In fact, if your kids have recess and are running around after they eat lunch, the concentrated sugar in the juice is much more likely to cause a stomachache than water.

Parents frequently ask,
"What do you think of sports drinks for kids?"

My Answer,
"I don't recommend them. Nonfat or 1% milk and water are by far the best."

There are *occasional* exceptions to this rule, depending on the child's activities. For example, if your child has 3 soccer games in one day and the weather is warm, then, yes ONE sports drink *may* be an appropriate choice (NOTE : that's one sports drink - not 3 or 4).

The truth is that sports drinks are really meant for athletes whose sporting activities are *long and vigorous* and, therefore, require quickly replenishing fluid and electrolytes lost from extensive sweating. **Companies have done a fabulous job marketing their beverages to the average adult and child, but they aren't the people who need sports drinks.**

With 3 boys who all love playing baseball, I've spent many hours at the baseball field. What I've seen is too many kids drinking Gatorade or other sports drinks that they definitely don't need. Some kids drink as many as 3 sports drinks in a two-hour game when their only activity has been occasionally running from first to second base or maybe from home plate to second base if they get a really good hit. That sprint didn't require a 20oz. sports drink. And the 125-375 calories they drank during that game is far greater than the calories they burned while playing, which involves a lot of standing in the field, sitting on the dugout bench and occasionally running the bases. This applies to most sports kids play, not just baseball. Yes, they need water. No, they don't need a sports drink. The bottom line is along with a few unneeded electrolytes, your child gets liquid sugar that increases the risk of tooth decay, excessive weight gain and obesity. Sounds like a bad deal to me!

So, if your child has one basketball, soccer or baseball game then water is the best way to stay hydrated. You can provide fruit as an after-game snack to get the same vitamins and electrolytes (potassium and sodium) that sports drinks contain. As a bonus, your child will get fiber, additional nutrients and less concentrated sugar from the fruit.

Energy Drinks . . . Let's take a minute to clarify the types of drinks available and what's in them.

Energy drinks contain substances, such as caffeine, guarana or taurine that work like stimulants in the body. **In May 2011 The American Academy of Pediatrics stated that** *energy drinks are never appropriate for children or adolescents.* They also stated that all caffeine-containing beverages, including soda, should be avoided because they can have harmful effects on a child's developing neurological and cardiovascular systems.

Sports drinks (which I've noticed many parents call energy drinks), have minerals, electrolytes and flavorings, in addition to sugar. They're designed to replace water and electrolytes that are lost during sweating with heavy exercise.

Vitamin drinks are flavored waters that have synthetic vitamins (usually Vitamin C and several B vitamins) added to them. Our diets are rarely deficient in these vitamins because they're found in many foods that we eat, so buying these waters for the added vitamins is a waste of money.

On the next page is a list of some popular energy drinks that should be avoided. (Note: this is not an all-inclusive list of all available energy drinks.)

Jill's Worst Picks :
Energy Drinks

Beverage	Size	Sugar (grams)	Calories	Caffeine (mg)	Sodium (mg)
Full Throttle	16 oz.	58	230	200	160
Java Monster	16 oz.	54	200	160	680
Java Monster Lo Ball*	16 oz.	12	100	135	460
Monster Energy	16oz.	54	200	160	360
Monster Energy Lo Carb*	16 oz.	6	20	135	360
Monster Extra Strength	12 oz.	38	160	160	300
Power Trip	16 oz.	52	200	210	380
Red Bull	12 oz.	39	160	114	140
Red Bull	16 oz.	52	220	154	200
Red Bull Sugar-free*	12 oz.	0	15	114	140
Rockstar Punched	16 oz.	62	260	240	110
Rockstar Energy Double Strength	16 oz.	62	280	160	80
Rockstar Sugar Free*	16 oz.	0	20	120	250
Rockstar Recovery	16 oz.	2	20	250	80
Go Girl	12 oz.	8	35	75	80
Go Girl Sugar-free*	12 oz.	0	< 5	100	100
Venom Energy	16.9 oz.	57	250	170	320
Venom Low Cal	16.9 oz.	6	60	170	320

Non Energy Drinks for comparison

Beverage	Size	Sugar (grams)	Calories	Caffeine (mg)	Sodium (mg)
Starbuck's Coffee (black)	16 oz.	0	5	330	0
Starbuck's Mocha	16 oz.	35	330	175	150
Soda (can)	12 oz.	38-51	140-195	0-54	30-75
Soda (bottle)	20 oz.	64-85	235-324	0-90	81-125

*contains artificial sweeteners

DID YOU KNOW . . .

Companies spend almost $500 million each year in advertising messages to children and adolescents about sugar-sweetened drinks?

When I look at the Nutrition Facts labels for juice, juice drinks, ice teas, sports drinks and other sweetened beverages, most are equally high in sugar when you compare them *ounce for ounce*. In other words, when you look at the sugar content for an equal serving size, most sweetened drinks have 3-4 grams of sugar per ounce. Below is a sampling of some of the many sweetened drinks.

Sugar-Sweetened Beverages

Beverage	Usual Serving	Total Sugar (grams)	Sugar per ounce
Soda (can)	12 oz.	38-51	3.2 -4.2g
Soda (bottle)	20 oz.	64-85	3.2 -4.2g
Juicy Juice	6.75 oz.	14	2.1g
Sobe	20 oz.	60	3g
Apple Juice	8 oz.	28	3.5g
Minute Maid	6.75 oz.	22-23	3.4g
Lemonade (can)	12 oz.	40	3.3g
Chocolate Milk	8 oz.	28	3.5g
Koolaid	6 oz.	19	3.2g
V8 Fusion	8 oz.	25	3.1g
AriZona Ice Tea	20 oz.	55	2.75g
Orange Juice	8 oz.	22	3.0g
Capri Sun	6 oz.	19	3.2g
Lemonade (pouch)	6 oz.	16	2.7
Snapple	16 oz.	36-40	2.2-2.5g
Gatorade	12-32 oz.	21-55	1.7g
Powerade	12-32 oz.	20-53	1.7g
Tomato Juice	8 oz.	8	1.0g

The take home message : your kids are much better off with a piece of fruit than *any* sweetened beverage, including 100% juice.

If you're going to offer sweetened drinks, 100% fruit juice is the best option, *and* make it a small serving (1/2 cup or 4 oz) to keep the sugar to a minimum.

Summing Up Beverages :

Fact # 1 : In the last 25 years the average soda sold in the United States has more than tripled in size from 6.5 oz. to 20 oz., increasing the amount of sugar from *5.5 teaspoons to 16 teaspoons* and the calories from *85 to 260 calories* with every soda!

Fact # 2 : Energy drinks are designed to rehydrate the body with fluid, sodium and potassium. A yogurt or piece of fruit + water can do as good a job, or better, at rehydrating your child.

Fact # 3 : Vitamin water provides synthetic vitamins, which does not work as effectively in our body as natural sources of vitamins and minerals. A piece of fruit + water provides a natural source of vitamins, along with other minerals and fiber, for greater nutrition that our body can really use.

Fact # 4 : Dairy products and some fruits provide a natural source of potassium, without the added sugar syrups found in sports drinks. Potassium is an important mineral that most kids don't get nearly enough of, so by choosing more fruits and dairy foods, your child will get a lot more of this important mineral.

Fact # 5 : Rarely do we need the sodium that is added to sports drinks. We get much more sodium in our diet than our bodies need, except for some athletes with long training days or kids participating in long, highly active sporting events.

Fact # 6 : A piece of fruit is healthier than a sweetened juice drink or 100% fruit juice.

The Bottom Line :

77% of Nutrition Experts give their children 2 cups of milk per day or more. 80% of Nutrition Experts allow soda not more than once a week. There's no benefit to sweetened beverages in your child's diet. There are many health benefits to helping your child get the recommended dairy servings each day! Eliminate sweet drinks from your grocery list and household to make a big, positive impact now on your child's diet and future health.

Your Game Plan :

Three examples of strategies to support your Game Plan…

1. I will buy a small reusable water bottle for my child's lunch bag.
2. I will buy only 100% juice and serve it 3 days or less per week.
3. I will talk to my family about drinking water and milk as our beverages.

What will you change about the beverages you offer your child? Will you change anything about the beverages you drink?

1. _____

2. _____

3. _____

Share Your Thoughts . . .

I would love to hear what changes you've made in the beverages you and your kids are drinking and if you have seen any benefits from making those changes. Are there any great tips or ideas you'd like to share?

**Please go to my website: www.400moms.com
or send me an e-mail at Jill@400moms.com
to share your thoughts and comments!**

CHAPTER 10

FAST FOOD & RESTAURANTS

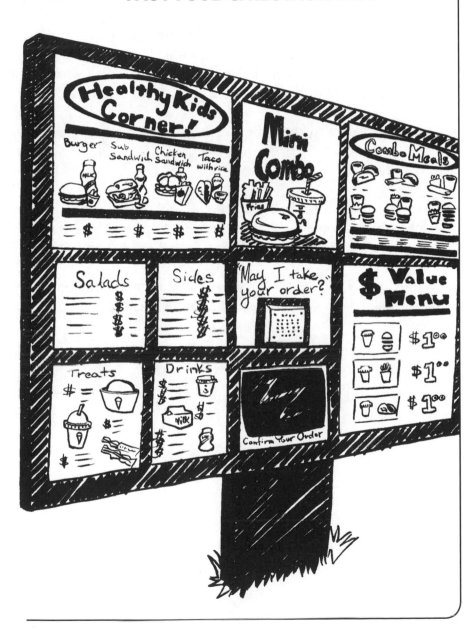

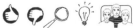

Eating On-The-Go : Fast-Food and Restaurants

Going out to eat can be a minefield of unhealthy options! A simple solution would be to never eat out. That way you would have complete control over your food choices, ingredients and amount of food served when you eat at home. But the reality is families are going to eat out because . . .

1. It's incredibly convenient in the fast-paced world we live in, and

2. Kids love it!

In this chapter I'll share the good, the bad and the ugly about the choices available to you. By the end of the chapter I hope you have more healthy choices, strategies and restaurants to encourage healthy eating for your child.

According to a report by the National Restaurant Association the typical American child aged 8 or older eats 4.2 commercially prepared meals each week.

When I asked Nutrition Experts about how many fast food meals their child eats per week, 80% reported once per week *or less.*

In other words, out of 21 meals most of these kids are eating no more than one fast food meal per week.

Another really important finding was that 1 out of 3 Nutrition Experts reported that their child ate fast food meals *0 times per week.*

FAST FOOD MEALS PER WEEK

Q: Why is there such a large discrepancy in how much fast food a Registered Dietitian's child eats compared to the average American child?

A: Because Nutrition Experts believe the harmful effects of too many fast food meals is not worth the convenience!

4.2x

**Typical
American
Child**

**1 or
Less**

**80% of
Nutrition Experts
Children**

None

**33% of
Nutrition Experts
Children**

Here's what too much eating out looks like to me:

TOO LITTLE	+	TOO MUCH	=	YOUR CHILD
FRUITS		FAT		LESS ENERGY
VEGETABLES		SUGAR		POOR CONCENTRATION
MILK		CALORIES		MORE SICK DAYS
FIBER				OBESITY
VITAMINS				DIABETES
MINERALS				HIGH CHOLESTEROL

If your child is eating a fast food meal once per week or less, it isn't likely to cause a health problem.

But, the simple truth is that if your child is eating take out, fast food or sit-down restaurant meals 4 or more times per week, like the average American child, then the chances for excessive weight gain and other serious health problems are very real!

Fast Food vs. Home Meal

Children who eat Fast Food consume **more calories, fat, sugar, and sugar-sweetened beverages**, along with **less fiber, milk, fruit and vegetables**.

Fast Food Meal:
HIGHER - Calories
HIGHER - Fat
HIGHER - Sugar
HIGHER - Sugar beverages

Meal From Home:
Fiber
Fruit
Vegetables
Milk

Children consume almost **twice as many calories** when they eat a restaurant meal compared to a meal at home. To make matters worse, they get more saturated fat, less fiber and less calcium. In other words, the healthy foods (milk, fruit and vegetables) get pushed out by the high fat meat, high fat starchy foods and high sugar drinks in the Fast Food or restaurant meal.

Yale's Rudd Center for Food Policy & Obesity evaluated 3,039 kids' meal combinations and found only 15 met the nutrition recommendations for a child's meal.

For example, a classic McDonalds Happy Meal with a hamburger, french fries and a soda is 590 calories, 34 grams of sugar and 20 grams of fat. The average preschooler needs about 1200 calories and 40 grams of fat daily. So you too can do the math and see that this *one meal provides half of the calories and fat* a preschooler needs for the whole day! Not only that, it provides all of the sugar and ¾ of the sodium a child should have daily. The reality is that if kids are eating this meal regularly, it's a prescription for excessive weight gain. How ironic that it's called a Happy Meal…I don't know about you, but it's not looking too happy to me.

So, What's a Mom to Do?

Eating dinner at home is the ideal option, but when you're in the midst of a hectic afternoon helping with homework and taking kids to activities, or a very busy day keeps you late at work, that take out or fast food restaurant becomes mighty appealing. And, thus, the reason fast food restaurants are on just about every corner.

Americans are eating out much more frequently than they did 20 years ago, and given our very busy lives, the convenience of eating out and buying commercially prepared meals is not going away. However, for the health of your kids, I strongly recommend you **limit fast food and take out meals to once/week**. If you currently eat out 3-4 times/week, I suggest you *gradually* change to more meals at home and fewer meals out. For example, start by having one more meal/week at home. After a month, add an additional quick meal at home. This gives you time to find quick, healthy options that work for you and your family. You can refer back to Chapter 5 for ideas.

As a busy Mom, I know the reality is that busy parents are going to buy take out and other restaurant meals some of the time, so the question is what are some healthier options that get dinner on the table quickly without being a nutrition bomb?

Finding a healthy, nutritionally-balanced meal in fast food restaurants is challenging, but there are a few choices you can make that are at least healthier than the standard meals.

Healthier Kid's Meal Combinations

If you find yourself at a fast food restaurant, the list below provides examples of "healthier" choices, but keep in mind a meal created at home will be the most nutritionally-balanced, or healthiest option.

"Healthier" Choices

#1: Subway Kids Meal Veggie Delite + Apple Slices + Low fat Milk

#2: KFC Grilled Chicken Breast + Corn on the Cob + Water

#3: Subway Kids Meal Roast Beef Mini Sub + Apples Slices + Low fat Milk

#4: KFC Grilled Chicken Drumstick + Corn on the Cob + Green Beans + Water

#5: Subway Kids Meal Turkey or Ham + Apple Slices + Low fat Milk

#6: Wendy's Jr. Hamburger + Mandarin Oranges + Low fat Milk

#7: Arby's Roast Beef Sandwich + Applesauce + Water

#8: McDonalds Chicken McNuggets + Apple Slices + 1% Milk

#9: McDonalds Hamburger + Apple Slices + 1% Milk

#10: Taco Bell Fresco Crunchy Taco + Mexican Rice + Water

The criteria I used to create this list is based on approximately 1/3 of the recommended calories, total fat and saturated fat per day for children.

It's important to note that the sodium in all of these meals is higher than the ideal amount of 400mg of sodium for a child's meal, and therefore aren't healthy, but are healthier than other choices. This is one of the many challenges with restaurant meals…they are simply too high in sodium, and there would be no options on the list if I used a recommended amount of sodium.

So I made a compromise: choose the healthiest meals with the least amount of sodium. The meals in the list range from 460mg to 790mg of sodium. Yet another reason to limit how often your child eats take-out, fast food and restaurant meals!

It's also important to note that menus in fast food restaurants can differ from one region of the country to another and that restaurants are frequently changing their menus, so all of the "Healthier Choices" may not be available in your area.

My recommendation is that you take time to review the nutrition information on the websites for the restaurants you most frequently visit.

The criteria I used to create the "Healthier Choices" list can be a guide when reviewing the nutrition information and help you determine which menu items are healthiest for your child.

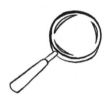

Nutrition Criteria for "Healthiest" Kids Meals:

< 450 Calories

< 15 grams Total Fat

< 5 grams Saturated Fat

< 1 gram Trans Fat

I know busy parents don't always have the time to review nutrition information, so in addition to now knowing some of the "Healthiest Kid Picks", another strategy is to pay close attention to the portion your child orders.

Portion sizes can make a big difference in how many extra calories your child eats or drinks.

Below are calorie comparisons of common "extras" at fast food restaurants. By having your child choose milk instead of soda and fruit instead of chips or French fries, you cut out 165 to 400 low quality calories. When your child chooses a smaller serving of dessert, he saves 100 to 500 calories of fat and sugar.

Fast Food Items	*Calories
8 oz. low fat Milk	100
6 oz. Juice Box	100
Small Soda	150
Large Soda	310
Subway Apple Slices	35
Wendy's Mandarin Orange Cup	90
1 oz. bag of Chips	150
2 oz. bag of Chips	300
Small French Fries	280
Large French Fries	500
McDonald's Vanilla Kiddie Cone	45
McDonald's Regular Vanilla Ice Cream Cone	150
Small Wendy's Chocolate Frosty	320
12 oz. McDonald's Vanilla Triple Thick Shake	420
16 oz. McDonald's Chocolate Triple Thick Shake	550

* *Calories vary according to flavor; therefore, average calculated*

Healthy Strategies When Eating Out

I believe it's important that children have some "say" in what they order when eating out. However, I also believe parents should help guide those choices.

Here are some tips to help you navigate the restaurant menus and steer your child toward healthier options :

1. **Allow your child to choose between 2 healthier menu items.**
   Example: "You can order the Grilled Chicken Sandwich or the Jr. Hamburger."

2. **Limit the number of unhealthy items to one, while still giving your child a choice.**
   Example: "You can order the kids' soda or the french fries, but not both."

3. **Prior to going to a restaurant, set the expectation of what choices will be acceptable.**
   Example: "Instead of french fries, you can choose salad, fruit or yogurt as your side dish."

4. **Improve the nutrition of the meal by ordering milk or water, instead of soda, lemonade or juice.**

5. **After milk or water, the next healthiest drink to choose is 100% fruit juice.**

6. **Choose grilled or baked entrees.**

7. **Avoid meats that are breaded, battered or batter-dipped.**

8. Avoid choices described as fried, creamy, crispy, scalloped, Alfredo, au gratin, cheese sauce or cream sauce.

9. Order salad for your child to eat with their pizza. This helps balance the meal and decreases the number of slices eaten.

10. In a sit-down restaurant, request a ½ order or "child's portion" of a healthier adult meal for your child.

11. If you have more than one child, instead of ordering from the kids menu, buy a healthier adult meal for them to share.

12. Ask for condiments on the side (mayonnaise, butter, sour cream, salad dressing, sandwich sauces) to control how much "extras" get added to your child's meal.

13. Purchase just the entrée "take out". Bring it home to combine with baby carrots (or other vegetable), fruit and milk for a quick meal.

14. Order thin crust pizza and keep the toppings to the healthiest options : cheese, vegetables, chicken and Candian bacon with pineapple.

15. Skip buffets. As you know, too many choices leads to too much food, whether you're a kid or an adult.

16. Share a dessert. If everyone really wants dessert, then share one (or two, depending on the size of your family), instead of everyone having their own.

Quick Meals at Home

Just like you, Nutrition Experts have very busy lives, juggling work and family, yet the number of meals eaten out is less than average. So what do they do to get food on the table quickly without buying fast food or restaurant meals regularly?

In addition to ideas in Chapter 5, here are some suggestions to try . . .

1. Frozen Entrees, such as chicken nuggets or fish sticks.
Bake them in the oven and combine them with cut up apples, baby carrots and milk. Kids love them and they're lower in fat than the fast food version....a win for you and a win for your kids!

2. Try Vegetarian Corn Dogs.
Kids love the outer batter, and they're much healthier than the traditional corn dog. Keep them on hand in the freezer, pop them in the toaster oven to cook and combine with fresh strawberries, steamed broccoli and milk for a quick, healthy meal.

3. Pasta with Marinara Sauce - cooks in 10 minutes.
Add some leftover chicken or frozen, pre-cooked turkey meatballs that can be heating while the pasta is cooking. The marinara sauce counts as a vegetable. Add a fruit and milk and dinner is served.

4. Frozen Bean Burritos (check the label; choose ones with no more than 10 grams Total Fat).
Pop them in the microwave, and, yes, you know the routine....add any fruit, vegetable and milk....dinner is done!

5. Frozen Skillet Meals.

I sometimes refer to these as "meals in a bag". Examples include Chicken Chow Mein, Beef & Broccoli, Garlic Shrimp and Chicken with Pasta. There are many brands, such as Trader Joe's, Bird's Eye Voila!, Newman's Own Complete Skillet Meal, Safeway Select Skillet Meal, Bertolli Meals for Two and Eating Right Complete Skillet Meal. The challenge with these meals is finding the healthy options. Some flavors are high in fat and most are high in sodium. Look for skillet meals with **no more than 10 grams fat and as close to 600mg of sodium per serving**.

6. Chicken Wrap

Using leftover chicken (or frozen, cooked grilled chicken breasts), chop chicken, then mix with chopped lettuce, tomatoes, cucumber and low fat Caesar, Ranch or Italian dressing. Spoon mixture onto a flour tortilla, roll and serve….with any fruit, vegetable and milk, of course.

NOTE: You can substitute sliced deli ham, roast beef or turkey for the leftover chicken. Mix the dressing with the vegetables, place the deli meat on the tortilla and spoon the lettuce mixture on top of the deli meat, then roll into a wrap.

7. Scrambled Eggs

With whole wheat toast, fruit, vegetable and milk. Done!

8. Crockpot Meals

There are MANY free recipes on the Internet that can be quickly assembled in the morning or the night before & refrigerated. Start the Crockpot in the morning and dinner is ready when you get home.

9. Store-Bought Rotisserie Chicken

Remove the skin, pat the meat with paper towels to remove as much extra fat as possible. Steam frozen vegetables, add unsweetened applesauce and milk.

10. Fast Tacos

Brown lean ground turkey or beef with onions (if your child will eat them), add taco seasoning and a can of beans, serve with taco shells or flour tortillas, salsa, shredded reduced-fat cheese, lettuce, tomatoes. Add fruit, raw vegetable and milk. Presto!

Advice From Moms Like You . . .

Do you ever wonder what other Moms do to get their kids to eat healthy restaurant meals? Here are 6 ways Moms just like you get their kids to make healthy restaurant choices:

1. Put Your Foot Down

"I have a conversation before going out to eat about what meals are acceptable choices. If my kids don't want those options, then we don't go out to eat."

"I give my kids a choice of healthier restaurants that I'm willing to take them to. If they don't like the choices, we don't go."

2. Use Incentives

"While on vacation I told my teenagers that whoever could go the whole week without eating fried foods would get 20 dollars at the end of the trip. It worked like a charm! It created a fun competition and helped them focus on making healthy choices. They both earned the 20 dollars."

3. Order from the Adult Menu

"Although it's more expensive, there are more healthy options, and we take the extra home to eat as leftovers."

4. The Lure of a Toy

"I tell my kids they can only get the toy that comes with the meal if they have fruit and milk instead of fries and soda."

5. Let Them Choose

"I let them choose whatever they want to eat, telling them it's a special occasion. Then we don't go again for several months."

6. Compromise

"I let them choose only one unhealthy item. They have to have a healthy sandwich, but can choose the small soda, chips, or fries, but only one of those options."

The Bottom Line :

Eat at home almost every night. By having quick meal options available in your cupboard and freezer, you can decrease how often your family eats out.

Your Game Plan :

Three examples to help your Game Plan work.

1. I will stock frozen entrees to have available for a quick meal.
2. I will talk to my family about decreasing how often we eat out to ___ nights/week.
3. I will talk to my kids about choosing low fat milk or water instead of soda when we eat out.

What will you do differently when it comes to eating fast food or in restaurants? Will you make quick-prep meals at home more often? Will you help your child make healthier choices when you eat out as a family? Or will you try some of the healthy strategies that other moms use? Write down 1-3 things you will change about eating-on-the-go.

1._____

2._____

3._____

Share Your Thoughts . . .

Please share what changes you've made around eating on-the-go. What benefits have come from making the change? Have you faced any challenges? Are there any great tips or ideas you'd like to share?

Please go to my website: www.400moms.com or send me an e-mail at Jill@400moms.com to share your thoughts and comments!

CHAPTER 11

PORTIONS

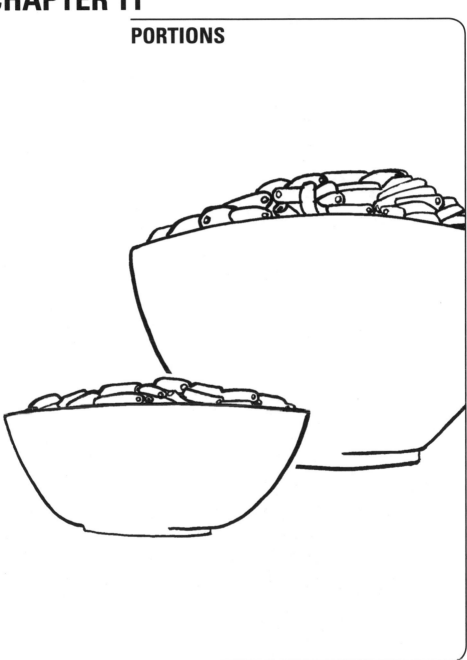

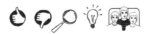

Portions . . . How Much Is Too Much?

I find parents are commonly confused by the terms "**portion**" and "**serving**", so I'll take a moment to differentiate what is a "portion" and what is a "serving".

A PORTION is the amount of food you choose to eat for a meal or snack.

A SERVING is a recommended, measured amount of food or beverage.

Serving sizes are determined by the USDA (United States Department of Agriculture) and the FDA (Food and Drug Administration).

Why Does It Matter?

The reason to distinguish the two terms is that many foods are packaged as a single portion, but contain several servings. For example, a box of macaroni and cheese is packaged as a single portion. But when you read the Nutrition Facts label it shows that the box contains 2 servings. This is important to pay attention to because the label will show calories and other nutrients for *one serving*, when, in fact, we usually eat the whole package or portion, which is two servings or more.

In the figure below, the Nutrition Facts label shows the serving size is 1 cup and contains 250 calories and 12 grams of total fat. But if your child eats the whole package as one portion, then it's 2 servings, so your child is actually eating 500 calories and 24 grams of total fat.

Macaroni and Cheese

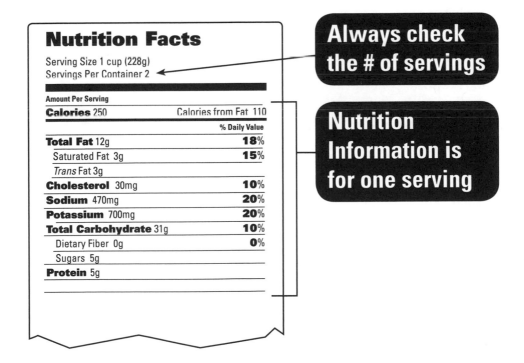

Nutrition Facts

Serving Size 1 cup (228g)
Servings Per Container 2

Always check the # of servings

Amount Per Serving

Calories 250   Calories from Fat 110

Nutrition Information is for one serving

	% Daily Value
Total Fat 12g	**18**%
Saturated Fat 3g	**15**%
Trans Fat 3g	
Cholesterol 30mg	**10**%
Sodium 470mg	**20**%
Potassium 700mg	**20**%
Total Carbohydrate 31g	**10**%
Dietary Fiber 0g	**0**%
Sugars 5g	
Protein 5g	

The take home message is . . .

By checking Nutrition Facts labels you won't be misled by what you think you're giving your child and what she is actually eating. **Be especially careful reading labels for sweetened drinks, snacks and desserts.**

For example, this 2 oz. bag of chips from the deli shows the serving size as 1 oz., or half the bag. But who eats ½ a bag? No one! So really your child is getting *double* the calories, fat and sodium in this portion size. Some products now list the nutrition information for the whole package. Not all labels will show this, though, so read the label carefully!

Another example is a serving of ice cream. The Nutrition Facts label shows a serving is ½ cup with 12 servings in the container. Do you ever get 12 servings out of your 1/2-gallon of ice cream? I don't think anyone does.

But I've found a strategy that works! First I buy light ice cream. Second, I bought a smaller ice cream scoop, so when my kids put 2 scoops of light ice cream in their bowl, it equals about ¾ cup ice cream, or 1 ½ servings instead of two. So my kids still get the "2 scoops" they like, but they're smaller scoops and, therefore, less calories, sugar and fat than if we used the traditional ½ cup ice cream scoop. Yes, they noticed the change, but after using the new scoop a few times, it became the routine. Give it a try.

Nutrition Facts

Serving Size 1oz.
Servings Per Container 2

Amount Per Serving

Calories 150	Calories from Fat 70
	% Daily Value
Total Fat 8g	**12%**
Saturated Fat 1.5g	**7%**
Trans Fat 0g	
Cholesterol 0mg	**0%**
Sodium 180mg	**7%**
Total Carbohydrate 17g	**6%**
Dietary Fiber 1g	**6%**
Sugars 1g	
Protein 2g	

Chips Label

Nutrition Facts

Serving Size 1/2 Cup
Servings Per Container 12

Amount Per Serving

Calories 140	Calories from Fat 25
	% Daily Value
Total Fat 3g	**4%**
Saturated Fat 2g	**9%**
Trans Fat 0g	
Cholesterol 10mg	**4%**
Sodium 30mg	**1%**
Total Carbohydrate 27g	**9%**
Dietary Fiber 0g	**1%**
Sugars 24g	
Protein 1g	

Light Ice Cream Label

In addition to multiple serving sizes in one package, there's the very big problem of portion sizes.

Over the past 25 years, the portion sizes of packaged foods and restaurant meals have grown significantly.

Most restaurant meals today range from 3 to 8 servings, and guess what? We eat all or almost all of what is served. That wouldn't be a problem if we then decreased our portions at other meals to "balance" the total calories we eat for the day. But the reality is, we eat the large portions and don't decrease our portions at the next meal or meals, so we end the day with a surplus of calories.

For example, when we eat a 4-ounce bagel at breakfast, we've already consumed 4 Grain Servings, which is most of what we need for the whole day. We then eat more Grain Servings at lunch and again at dinner, far exceeding what is recommended. When this pattern is repeated for days, then weeks and months, weight gain is inevitable.

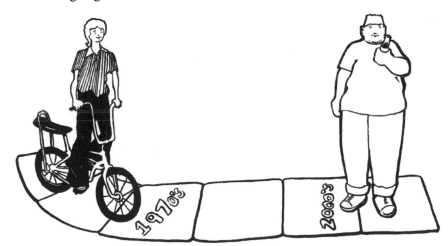

About 32% of American kids are overweight or obese today, compared with 5% in the early 1970's.

I've talked about several likely causes for this weight gain trend, including consuming too many sweetened drinks and too many high fat, high sugar snacks and desserts. Another likely cause is the expanding portion sizes over the last 25 to 30 years. As the portions have increased in size, so have our bellies!

The phenomenon of ever-expanding portion sizes has been described as "Portion Distortion".

The National Heart, Lung and Blood Institute is a government agency that has developed a quiz and educational materials to increase awareness about how our portions have changed over the years.

The problems created by excessive portions are numerous and sometimes subtle.

Problem #1:

Large portions are "normal". Kids today have developed a distorted view of what is a normal portion. When I was a child, a muffin was 1 ½ to 2 ounces and was baked in a small muffin tin. Today, a muffin is 4 ounces and made in a much larger muffin tin. The 4-ounce muffin has become a "normal" portion to our kids because large muffins are all they've ever seen and eaten.

Problem #2:

Eating large portions pushes out valuable nutrients. Kids are filling up on large portions of low-nutrient foods (snacks, desserts and sweetened drinks), instead of filling up on nutrient–dense foods, such as fruits, vegetables and whole grain foods.

Problem #3:

Staying at a healthy weight becomes near impossible. With time, the extra calories from large portion sizes can't be used up with activity so the extra calories get stored as fat and excessive weight.

The Calorie Consequences of Portion Distortion

I've included several examples comparing food portions and calories from 25 years ago to portions today. The calorie difference is striking and helps explain why it's so difficult to manage our weight when the calorie surpluses are so large.

COMPARISON OF PORTIONS	25-Years Ago		Today		LOOK AT THE DIFFERENCE
	Portion	Calories	Portion	Calories	Calorie Surplus
Bagel	3-inch	140	6-inch	350	210
Blueberry Muffin	1.5 ounces	210	4 ounces	500	290
Cheeseburger	1	330	1	590	260
French Fries	2.4 ounces	210	6.9 ounces	610	400
Soda	6.5 ounces	82	20 ounces	250	168
Spaghetti w/ 3 Meatballs	1 cup sauce	500	2 cups sauce	1020	520
Chocolate Chip Cookie	½ ounce	60	4 ounces	500	440

Source: National Heart, Lung and Blood Institute, National Institutes of Health.

To learn more and take the Portion Distortion quiz, go to:
http://hp2010.nhlbihin.net/portion

Portion Size 25-Years Ago

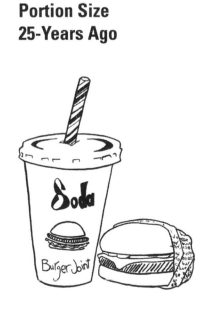

Portion Size Today

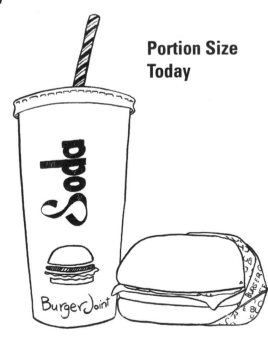

A Real Life Scenario . . .

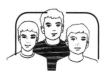
One night my kids were having dessert after dinner and one of my boys was scooping low-fat ice cream into his bowl. As he was about to dish up a second scoop, I said, "Oh, one scoop is the right amount. What you have in your bowl is a serving of ice cream." His jaw dropped and he said, "WHAT! Nobody eats *that much* ice cream! That's ridiculous; it's *so* small! "

I then pointed out that what he had in his bowl was ½ cup, which is the serving size listed on the Nutrition Facts label and the amount recommended for "extras" or "sweets". Twenty-five years ago 1/2 cup is exactly what would have been served, but today it seems ridiculously small when we're used to seeing 1 to 1 ½ cups of ice cream served. A classic example of Portion Distortion!

When Portion Distortion happens in our home, I take the opportunity to remind my kids what an "ideal" or "healthy" portion is versus a "typical" portion they see daily.

This strategy of reestablishing a realistic portion size is one way to deal with **Problem #1: Large portions are normal.**

As a matter of fact, it addresses **Problem #2 (Eating large portions pushes out valuable nutrients)** and **Problem #3 (Staying at a healthy weight becomes near impossible)** as well.

What Do You Do When . . .

Your child comes home after school and is ready for a snack. She grabs the box of crackers from the cupboard, reaches in and pulls out a heaping fistful, then sits down at the computer with the box nearby. I've seen this at my house, for sure!

There are several ways you could choose to intervene. Below are several examples of what you could say to your child.

#1: "That looks like more than one serving of crackers."

You then ask your child to look at the Nutrition Facts label to see what is listed as a serving size. Once she tells you the serving size, you can suggest she eat the amount listed as a "serving", and if she's still hungry, offer a fruit, yogurt or other healthy choice. This approach teaches your child how to read the Nutrition Facts label and helps her learn about serving sizes.

#2: "Please put your crackers in a bowl, and then put the box back in the cupboard."

This is a useful approach to help control the total portion your child eats, but doesn't address how many servings she actually ate.

#3: "Please sit down at the table to eat your snack before using the computer."

This strategy teaches your child to pay attention to what and how much she is eating in the moment. Eating while distracted is what I call "unconscious eating" where we lose track of how much we've eaten and whether we're still hungry or full. The end result is eating more food than was really needed to meet our hunger needs. By sitting at the table and doing nothing but eating, your child pays attention to hunger and fullness cues and enjoys the food she is eating in the moment.

Visualize The Healthy Plate . . .

Numerous studies have shown that the more food you put in front of someone, the more they eat.

In one study people were given different size sandwiches on four different occasions, ranging from a 6-inch sandwich up to a 12-inch sandwich. The results? Participants ate significantly more as the sandwich size got larger. This result has been shown in several other studies as well when participants were served increasing portions of pasta, soup or snack foods. What appears to happen is that people *unknowingly* eat more when presented with more food.

Interestingly, similar studies have been done with children and have shown the same behavior: eating greater amounts as portions get larger. One study with preschoolers, however, showed that the 3 ½ year-olds did not overeat the larger portions, but the 5-year-olds did, suggesting that as children get older they may lose the ability to adjust food intake when larger portions are served.

Given the results of these studies, it's just as important to control portions when eating *at home* as it is when eating in a restaurant.

You might be wondering "How do I control portions?" One surefire way is to become an expert at estimating serving sizes!

Not only can you teach your child about healthy choices, but also about realistic serving sizes for meals, snacks, beverages and desserts. At times it may feel like you're paddling upstream, against a river of "super" sizes, "king" sizes and "value" sizes, but with time and repetition your child will learn the difference between the amount restaurants and food companies provide and what his body really needs.

One useful strategy for serving appropriate portions is to "visualize" the recommended amounts to serve. When you serve an accurate amount, your child is learning how much should be on her plate.

So how do you "visualize" the portions? One strategy I've recommended for years is to use the Healthy Plate Model to determine how much food to serve. I talked about this concept in Chapter 5 and here is a reminder of what it looks like :

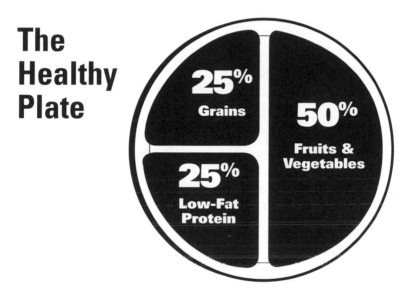

By visualizing this plate, you will remember to cover ½ the plate with fruits and vegetables, leaving ¼ of the plate for protein and ¼ of the plate for the grain/starch choice.

With younger children, use a smaller plate, which will help adjust the portions for a smaller stomach. With teenagers, an adult plate will be more realistic for their appetite and you can fill it with larger amounts of the same food groups.

You might notice that my example of The Healthy Plate is slightly different than the ChooseMyPlate recommendation, which has a little larger amount of vegetables than fruit on the plate. Since I've seen many people have success with this simple visual over the years, I'm sticking with it. Simple is always good!

DOWNSIZING PORTIONS
for the whole family

Out of Sight, Out of Mind...

- Serve a reasonable portion on individual plates, instead of leaving serving dishes on the table. When food is easily accessible, we are more likely to eat extra.

- Immediately put leftovers away. After serving each person, put leftovers in the refrigerator. The less food we see, the less we are likely to eat.

- Freeze leftover treats and then thaw only the amount for single servings. Relying on willpower to avoid eating extras doesn't work for kids or adults.

- Store tempting foods in the back of cupboards and up high. The less accessible they are, the less often they will be eaten.

Measuring Know-How...

- Weigh or measure a portion (i.e. ½ cup rice or a 3 oz. chicken breast) to see how it fits on your plate; with practice you will be able to "eyeball" or visualize the correct portion to serve each person without having to measure each time.

- Measure snacks, desserts, entrees and starchy foods; allow extras of fruits and vegetables.

- Measure the amount of beverage and note how high it fills your glass or a child's cup. Now you know how much to pour each time to serve the right amount.

- Use smaller plates, bowls and cups. We like to fill our plate or bowl, so using smaller dishes allows us to have a full plate and not feel like we're getting cheated.

- Buy single portions of snack foods or divide the large package into several smaller containers or baggies to serve as single servings for snacks or in a lunch bag.

Successful Substitutions...

- Change the candy bowl to a bowl of fruit.

- Provide fruit or vegetables as your child's 2nd helping.

- Serve your child's snack in a bowl instead of allowing him to eat out of the bag or box.

- Eating a healthy snack between meals can help avoid excessive hunger before a meal and prevent snacking before the meal or overeating at mealtime.

Eating Behaviors...

- **Eliminate distractions.** Have you ever been eating and watching TV and suddenly looked down and the food was gone without realizing you had eaten it? When you and your kids are eating, just eat! Sit down at the table, talk about the day, and focus on the meal. Avoid watching TV, reading, texting, working on the computer or doing other things while eating. It's easy to overeat when your attention is focused on something else.

- **Slow Down.** Eating more slowly allows the body to signal it's full, which can decrease second helpings and prevent feeling "stuffed" afterwards.

- **Wait 20 minutes** before having a 2nd helping. It's difficult to get some kids to slow down while eating the meal, so having a family "rule" that you wait 20 minutes before having seconds accomplishes the same thing...allowing the body time to signal it's full. If your child is still hungry after waiting, then another helping is ok.

Visualize It . . .

In addition to picturing The Healthy Plate when you're serving a meal, many parents like visual examples for specific amounts and types of food. Below are examples of common measurements and an object to help you picture and remember what that amount looks like.

Standard Measurement:

½ cup
1 cup
1 ounce
3 ounces of meat or chicken
3 ounces of fish
1 teaspoon
1 Tablespoon
2 Tablespoons

Is the size of . . .

½ of a baseball
A woman's fist
A golf ball
A deck of cards
A checkbook
Tip of your thumb
A poker chip
A golf ball

Recommended Serving:

1 medium potato
1 small apple
1 "serving" of vegetables
1 "serving" of salad
1 "serving" of fruit salad
1 burrito
1 ear of corn
2 oz. muffin or biscuit
1 Tablespoon salad dressing
1 Tablespoon butter or mayonnaise
1 ½ oz. cheese
2 oz. bagel
1 "serving" of ice cream
¼ cup nuts or raisins

Is the size of . . .

A computer mouse
A baseball
½ baseball
A woman's fist
½ baseball
Checkbook length
8-inch pencil length
A hockey puck
1 capful from bottle of salad dressing
1 poker chip
4 dice
A can of tuna
½ baseball
A large egg

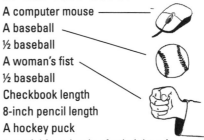

If your child is overweight, it may be necessary to decrease the total amount you're serving, in addition to accurately estimating serving sizes. There are several ways you can downsize portions without leaving everyone hungry.

The Bottom Line :

Portions are way out of control! They're distorting what our kids think is a healthy amount to eat and contributing to excessive weight gain for kids and adults.

Your Game Plan :

Three examples of strategies to help your Game Plan…

1. I will buy smaller plates to use at dinner.
2. I will buy extra fruit and vegetables so I can serve ½ the plate fruits & veggies at dinner.
3. I will take the Portion Distortion quiz with my kids.

What changes will you make to help your child understand what a normal or healthy portion looks like? What will you do differently to prevent Portion Distortion?

1._____

2._____

3._____

Share Your Thoughts . . .

Tell me about the changes you've made in the portions you buy or serve to your child. What benefits have you seen from making these changes? Have you had any challenges with what you've tried? Are there any great tips or ideas you'd like to share?

**Please go to my website: www.400moms.com
or send me an e-mail at Jill@400moms.com
to share your thoughts and comments!**

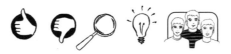

CHAPTER 12

WHAT NOW?

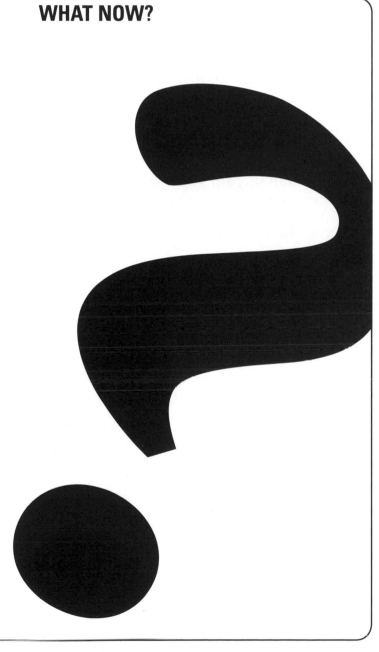

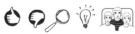

What Now?

Congratulations! You've made it to the final chapter of the book! Being the last chapter, it begs the question, *"What now?"*

What will be different about the way you feed your kids?

What foods will you stock in your cupboards?

Will the food in your refrigerator be healthier now?

What healthy changes will you and your family continue for the long-term?

It's important to acknowledge that even Nutrition Experts are not perfect in the way they feed their kids. There's always room to improve our own food and health habits, as well as the habits we teach our kids.

Just like Nutrition Experts, you need to choose what's most important to focus on when it comes to healthy eating and then *be consistent* in what you say and do. The expression "you have to pick your battles", applies to healthy eating, just as it applies to other areas of our lives.

For example, in my survey a few Registered Dietitians (about 6%) reported that their kids eat high sugar cereals for breakfast.

Although I didn't specifically ask these Nutrition Experts why they provided high-sugar cereals, my guess is they've decided it's important to eat a high fiber cereal, even if it's higher in sugar. Or maybe they believe that having breakfast is more important, even if it's a sweetened cereal, than no breakfast at all. Or maybe avoiding high sugar cereals isn't "worth the battle", but serving lots of fruits and vegetables is "worth the battle" to them.

My survey also revealed that 1 out of every 6 Nutrition Experts serve a sweet snack daily. You might be surprised that some Nutrition Experts allow sweets that often. But maybe the sweet snack is portion-controlled or one of the healthier sweet snack options. In that case it becomes an "extra" that is balanced with the many healthy choices their child eats throughout the day. It can also serve as an example that there are no "bad" foods and that all foods can be part of a healthy diet if they're eaten in moderation and balanced with mostly healthy choices.

So what is my point?

No need to aim for perfection.
Instead, choose healthy eating goals that are achievable for your kids, realistic for your family and improves their health.

Just as Nutrition Experts choose components of healthy eating they believe are the most important to emphasize, I recommend you choose 2 or 3 areas to focus on with your kids.

At the end of each chapter I summed up the information with the most important message, referred to as *The Bottom Line.* When faced with lots of information, ideas and strategies, it often helps people move forward and decide what their next step will be when the most important information is summarized.

So, what's the summary message for the entire book?

For the first time in United States history, the current generation is expected to live *shorter* lives than their parents.

You can help your child beat these odds by providing the BEST diet for kids:

THE BOTTOM LINE . . .

The BEST diet for your child is :

B = Breakfast every day

E = Eat 5 or more fruits and vegetables every day

S = Stop Sodas and Sweet Drinks

T = Trim down Fast Food & Portion Sizes

If you do these 4 things consistently, you help your child avoid obesity, high cholesterol, high blood pressure and Type 2 diabetes now and as he or she reaches adulthood!

What a gift to give your child!

Creating a Healthy America

As you work to improve your family's food habits, you're also part of a bigger movement to shift the tide of obesity and chronic disease in our country. We *can* create a healthier America, one child and one family at a time. I believe there are several important factors that must be in place before a Healthy America becomes a reality.

Fact # 1 : Americans must take responsibility!

What I'm talking about here is being conscious about our purchasing behaviors. We need to take responsibility for what we're buying at the grocery store and in restaurants, for ourselves and our kids. If we, as consumers, stop purchasing soda and sweet drinks, demand healthier snacks for our kids and request smaller restaurant meals, companies will respond.

Have you noticed the Trans-fat in most snacks and desserts is gone? That's because companies responded when there was enough pressure and the threat of decreased sales. If we stop buying cereals loaded with sugar and instead purchase high fiber, low sugar cereals, companies will make more of what we want and are buying. If we go to the fast food restaurants that offer healthier options, instead of going to restaurants that serve 1200-calorie meals, then more restaurants will improve what they offer on their menus. If we stop buying the out-of-control portions or begin sharing meals when eating out, restaurants will follow our lead and make changes to their meal sizes.

Secondly, we need to take responsibility for *how many* meals we eat out. It's true that our lives are very busy and that's not likely to change in the near future. But the reality is we cannot continue to eat restaurant meals 3 to 5 times/week as most families currently do and expect that kids and parents will be a healthy weight. There are ways to prepare quick meals at home that have far fewer calories and are much healthier than what we get when eating out.

It will require Americans taking responsibility for what they choose to buy and how often they eat out before we'll see a shift toward healthier options and portion sizes.

Fact # 2 :
Americans must move more!

The list of health benefits from exercise is phenomenal! I wasn't going to list them, but decided I must because there are over 20 benefits, many of which are pretty compelling. They range from lowering cholesterol to boosting moods and energy.

Here are the many benefits of exercise:

- Increases Energy
- Prevents or improves Type 2 Diabetes
- Improves Mood
- Increases Muscle Strength
- Live Longer
- Improves digestion
- Weight Management
- Helps Prevent Osteoporosis
- Lowers Triglycerides
- Increases Metabolism
- Helps Prevent some types of Cancer

- Improves Memory
- Improves Sleep
- Improves Concentration
- Decreases Stress
- Helps Prevent Back Pain
- Lowers Blood Pressure
- Decreases Anxiety
- Improves Depression
- Lowers Cholesterol
- Improves School Performance

It's true that many of the health benefits listed are a result of doing sustained aerobic activity, such as brisk walking. However, I also want to emphasize the importance of being more active within our daily lives.

Over the past 50-years our activity levels have dropped dramatically. Our lives have become so automated that it takes very little physical effort to do our daily tasks. This puts us at a huge disadvantage (no pun intended) when it comes to managing weight because the food calories we eat quickly surpass how many calories our body burns each day.

So we have a double whammy going on here: larger portions providing extra food calories (calories IN) combined with less calorie burning from daily activity (calories OUT).

Think about all the opportunities we have to sit: commuting to and from school, sitting at a desk all day, driving to and from activities, playing video or handheld games and sitting in front of the TV or computer after school. It can add up to more than 14 hours of sitting each day.

We must figure out ways to incorporate more movement into our day by making a conscious effort to break up all the sitting time.

Here are some ideas to get your family moving more :

- take the stairs instead of the elevator

- park farther away from your destination

- walk your dog (or a neighbor's dog)

- walk to do nearby errands

- have your kids help with housework and yard work

- wash the car together

- play at the playground

- play frisbee at the park

- play indoor volleyball with a balloon

- buy a hoola hoop or jump rope for your child

- go for a bike ride

- walk around while talking on the phone

You may be thinking 10-15 minutes of moving won't do much, but the reality is that if your kids consistently stack enough small activity segments together throughout the day, they can burn an extra 200 calories or more, and weight management becomes much more achievable.

For more information about how many calories you burn for different activities, check this website: www.healthstatus.com/calculate/cbc

For more ideas of how to get short bursts of activity, check this website: www.abeforfitness.com

Being more active really can make a difference in weight and long-term health, even if it's not structured exercise.

Did you know . . .
Kids need at least 60 minutes of activity every day? This includes activities that are moderate to vigorous, like basketball or swimming, but also includes play time.

Playing tag outdoors, throwing a Frisbee, riding a bike, raking leaves or dancing to music all count toward activity.

Setting limits on screen time (TV, computer, video and handheld games) at home can free up time to be more active on school days and weekends. If parents would require that **homework and activity** are finished before any screen time is allowed each day, then kids would be much more likely to reach an hour of activity daily.

The Reward Trap . . .

Be careful not to allow your kids to fall into the trap of "eating back" the calories they just burned while exercising.

For example, I've seen many kids drinking a sports drink after a game. If they play for 30 minutes and drink a 20 oz. Gatorade afterwards, then they've just consumed 125 of the 150 calories they burned.

Or if they eat that chocolate chip cookie after the game they're sabotaging their exercise efforts because the cookie costs more in calories than what they burned in 30-minutes of play.

So be careful not to reward exercise efforts with food.

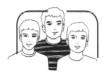
Over and over again I've seen the same Reward Trap with kids' activities and snacks. When my boys played soccer in elementary school, after every 30-minute game parents felt compelled to provide a juice bag, cookies, cupcakes, doughnuts or any other variety of junk food. Why does the reward for playing a game need to be junk food? How about a "high five" or a "great job, you really played hard!" The Energy In from the after-game snack often exceeds the amount of Energy Out from the minutes of actual activity each child plays. And what message are we sending to our kids when junk food is provided after every game?

If any snack is provided after a game it should be water and a piece of fruit. Then the message we send to our kids is that the body needs to be rehydrated and refueled with healthy choices after activity, not rewarded with junk food.

The Positive Domino Effect

In my nutrition consulting practice I've found that many people who exercise experience what I call a "Positive Domino Effect": when people are exercising, they're also more likely to be eating healthy foods. For example, clients tell me that if they exercise in the morning, they're more likely to eat a healthy breakfast afterwards, or if they exercise after work, they're more likely to eat a healthy snack in the afternoon and a healthy dinner.

The opposite effect is called "The Negative Spiral". When exercise stops, healthy food choices decline. The long term effect can be that stopping exercise leads to greater food calories and weight gain, which leads to even less exercise and more weight gain.

The Negative Spiral

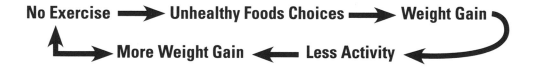

No Exercise ➞ Unhealthy Foods Choices ➞ Weight Gain

More Weight Gain ⬅ Less Activity

The heavier kids get, the harder it is for them to run, play games on the playground and climb stairs, so the natural tendency is for them to move less and continue to gain more weight. Not a good thing.

Fact # 3 :
We must get the junk out of our schools!

Parents need to step up and demand that schools provide a healthy environment for their children. A healthy environment addresses not just healthy meals on the breakfast and lunch menus, but also snacks sold during or after school, food given in class, and fundraisers.

You are your child's advocate, so insist that your child's school stops selling unhealthy snacks, such as doughnuts, chips and candy. Schools also need to stop supporting fundraisers that promote unhealthy choices by selling items such as cookie dough and chocolate. At the very least, you can be consistent with your message to provide healthy choices by not participating in these fundraisers and explaining to your child why you won't participate. If enough parents don't participate, the school will find other ways to raise money.

Another frequent source of junk food can be teachers, believe it or not! Handing out candy as a reward for good work or behavior needs to stop. First of all, food as a reward is not a healthy behavior. Secondly, there are many non-food items that can be provided as incentives that kids enjoy. There are a couple of ways you can address this issue. You can talk with your child's teacher about ways to decrease in-class junk food, provided by teachers or by parents. Teachers can create a policy and distribute it to parents at the beginning of the year establishing what foods are acceptable to bring for celebrations. You can also start or join your school's Wellness Committee and gradually work to establish a school-wide policy that promotes healthy choices for menus, snacks, parties, vending machines and fundraisers.

Until we provide the healthy choices kids need *at school and at home*, obesity will continue to be a major challenge for our kids.

Fact # 4 :
Calories must be posted on restaurant menus and menu boards.

In 2010 New York passed a state law requiring all restaurants to post the calories for each menu item. Not hidden in a brochure or inconveniently tucked away on a website, but posted right where you can actually read how many calories are in what you're about to order.

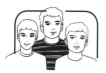 I was on vacation in New York with my family, and it was a great learning experience for all of us to have the calories front and center. The most shocking learning opportunity was at a baseball game at Yankee Stadium. My kids went with their Dad to the concessions to choose what to have for dinner. My oldest son chose a Sausage Dog (yes, a dietitian's nightmare!); my second son got a Soft Pretzel, and my youngest son chose Cheese Pizza. My oldest son came back to his seat and said, "Mom, you won't believe it! My sausage has less calories than the Soft Pretzel!" I was even more shocked than my son that a sausage could have fewer calories than a soft pretzel, and I'm a Nutrition Expert!

If a Nutrition Expert doesn't know all the calories in the menu choices, how will parents have any clue how many calories are in the foods their kids are eating?

California and Oregon have passed similar laws and The Affordable Care Act that was passed in 2010 included a requirement that all restaurant chains in the U.S. with greater than 20 establishments post nutrition information on their menus. The Food and Drug Administration has to propose the specific regulations and with possible legal battles, it could be years before we see calorie information in restaurants throughout the country.

It will be a real setback if legal battles or legislative changes end in favor of no calorie information being posted on menus.

Some of the questions being asked are :

Will calories on menus influence and improve consumer choices? Would consumers rather not be bothered with calorie information when they're trying to enjoy their meal?

Our experience while vacationing in New York was that having calorie information on the menus definitely increased my kids' awareness about what they were eating and helped me make healthier choices while eating out. Once again it comes back to taking responsibility.

If Americans (young and old) are going to manage their weight and be healthy, then having this information is critical. Rather than *guessing* what might be a healthy menu choice, the answer is available. Having the calorie information won't stop people from eating out, but it might influence what they choose and possibly how often they eat out.

And if consumers are "bothered" by knowing the calories in their choices when they're trying to enjoy their meal, they should be! Continuing to ignore the fact that excessive portions and calories are contributing to serious health problems for kids and adults is irresponsible!

It's time to take action!

Fact # 5 :
Whole, unprocessed foods rule.

Did you know that many of the children in our country are simultaneously *overweight* and *undernourished*? How can that be? When bodies are filled with highly processed foods containing artificial ingredients, lots of calories in a small serving and little or no nutrients (such as chips, candy, cookies, snack foods and sweet drinks), the body is starving for nutrients while getting excessive calories.

The nutrients most commonly deficient in a child's diet include calcium, fiber, folate, iron, magnesium, potassium and vitamin E. Where can you find most of these nutrients? Dairy, fruits, vegetables and whole grains. That's why whole, unprocessed foods rule.

We also know that foods in their natural form have greater health benefits because the nutrients in whole foods are better absorbed and utilized than the nutrients taken individually. There are substances present in whole foods that help us utilize all the valuable parts of the food.

Give your child's body what it really wants and needs: more fresh fruits, vegetables and whole grains instead of highly processed snacks, meals and desserts.

Fact # 6 :
Improved Nutrition Facts labels
are a must

Naturally-occurring sugar, sugar alcohols* and added sugar are lumped into the category of "Sugar" on the current Nutrition Facts label.

It isn't right that candies, such as jelly beans, Skittles or gummy worms are labeled with the same sugar content as raisins!

Although it's true that they both have about 17 grams of sugar per ounce, the source of sugar is entirely different: naturally-occurring fructose and glucose in raisins (along with fiber and important vitamins and minerals) vs. corn syrup, sugar, glucose syrup and confectioner's glaze in the candies.

A much more helpful Nutrition Facts label would list the amount of naturally-occurring sugar and added sugars separately.

It's worth pointing out that many companies have chosen to voluntarily list some types of fats separately on the Nutrition Facts Label (i.e. trans-fat, mono-unsaturated fat and polyunsaturated fat) when it works to their advantage. For example, when companies reformulated snacks to eliminate trans-fats, then they were willing to show the fats individually in order to use it as a marketing advantage. It's time to have transparency about what's really in the foods we're buying, so we can make educated choices.

When a cereal has fruit in it, we can't determine how much of the sugar in these cereals is from the fruit and how much is added sugar.

Knowing how much of the 17 grams of sugar in Raisin Bran or 9 grams of sugar in Special K with Berries is from the fruit would allow us to accurately compare these cereals with other healthy cereals that don't contain fruit. Until the labels are improved, the best option is to buy low-sugar cereals that don't contain fruit and add the fruit yourself.

*If a company makes a claim about a product, such as "No Added Sugar", then the sugar alcohol must be listed separately from sugar on the Nutrition Facts label. But if there are no claims made, then sugar alcohols can be listed as part of the total sugar.

Fact # 7 :
Moms MUST put themselves FIRST!

You might be thinking, "How is this important for a Healthy America?" It's very important because Moms are the ones who make things happen! Although many more dads are helping with the shopping and cooking for the household, Moms are still the primary managers or "gatekeepers" of food for the family. Moms determine *what* food comes into the house, *how much* of which foods are available, what restaurants the family goes to and what meals are served at home. Managing the shopping, meal planning and preparation is a really important job. When it comes to a Healthy America, Moms are the solution! The only way Moms can do this job well is if they're taking care of themselves *first,* so they have the energy and ability to help their families do the same.

I see too many Moms "Running on Empty": exhausted, irritable and feeling like things are out of control.

When your "tank is empty", it's difficult to provide what your kids and family need to be healthy. What do I mean by "taking care of you"?

#1. Get exercise   In order to be healthy and manage stress, this is a must! Not only are you modeling healthy behaviors or "walking the walk", but you'll also have more patience, more energy and likely better focus when you're exercising regularly. Patience, energy and focus will help you meet your family's needs a whole lot better.

#2. Take time for you   Doing something that is just for you is really important when your energy and time are regularly consumed by family needs. When you're feeling drained or depleted, it's near impossible to "be there" for your family. Taking time to "fill your tank" allows you to give your energy to meet your family's needs.

#3. Get Support   Don't try to "do it all" yourself. Over time, there's a "chipping away" effect where oftentimes weight increases, stress builds up and ultimately your health suffers. In order to find time to exercise and take time for you, you need a team! Make a list of all the people who can be a part of your team: your children, spouse, grandparents, neighbors, friends, other Moms, a personal trainer or coach. Then make a list of *how* these people can be of help to you. Finally, talk to them and get them on board with being your support, just as you support them! The bottom line is that when you take care of yourself, you take better care of your kids too.

What To Look For

The next few pages are a summary of all the "what to look for" guidelines, recipes, and important charts I've provided throughout the book to help you make the healthiest choices for your child. They're listed here as your quick, "go-to" guide.

Cereal:	6 grams of sugar or less 3 grams of fiber or more
Frozen Waffles:	6 grams of sugar or less 3 grams of fiber or more 5 grams of total fat or less
Crackers:	"3 & 3" Rule 3 grams of total fat or less 3 grams of fiber or more
Snack Bars:	5 grams of total fat or less 2 grams of fiber or more 8 grams of sugar or less
Yogurt (6oz.) :	20% Calcium or more 20% Vitamin D or more 20 grams of sugar or less
Dinner Meal:	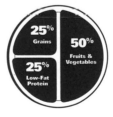
Fast Food Meal:	450 calories or less 15 grams Total Fat or less 5 grams Saturated Fat or less 0-1 gram Trans Fat
Desserts:	150 calories or less 2 grams saturated fat or less Limit sweets to once/day

Quick Reference Guide

Recipes

Quick Reference Guide

"Go-To" Guide Charts

Quick Reference Guide

Best Picks & Worst Picks

Cereal:	Worst Picks	page 26
	Best Picks	page 27
	Best High Fiber/Low Sugar	page 28
Crackers:	Best Picks	page 48
	Worst Picks	page 49
Yogurt:	Best Picks	page 52
Snack Bars:	Best Picks	page 55
	Worst Picks	page 56
Cookies:	Worst Picks	page 73
	Worst Picks	page 152
	Best Picks	page 153
Frozen Desserts:	Worst Picks	page 154, 155
	Best Picks	page 156, 157
Energy Drinks:	Worst Picks	page 178

Quick Reference Guide

Organic vs. Non-Organic Produce

Buy Organic: **(Highest Pesticide Risk)**	**Non-Organic:** **(Lowest Pesticide Risk)**
Apples	Sweet Potatoes
Celery	Corn
Bell Peppers	Pineapple
Peaches	Avocado
Strawberries	Cabbage
Nectarines (imported)	Peas
Grapes	Asparagus
Spinach	Mango
Lettuce	Eggplant
Cucumbers	Kiwi
Blueberries	Cantaloupe
Potatoes	Green Beans
Grapefruit	Mushrooms
Kale/Dk. Greens	Watermelon
	Onions

Source: The Environmental Working Group: www.ewg.org

Quick Reference Guide

Healthy Fat Choices For Your Child

Healthy fats are important for kids because they provide energy and help certain nutrients get absorbed and utilized by the body. The fats listed below are low in saturated fat, making them the healthiest choices for your child.

Olives

Avocado

Nuts: Almonds, Peanuts, Walnuts, Cashews, Pecans

Seeds: Sunflower, Pumpkin, Sesame

Peanut Butter

Almond Butter

Soy Nut Butter

Wheat Germ

Oils: Olive, Canola, Peanut, Sesame

Salad dressings made with oil (Italian, Vinaigrettes, Honey Dijon)

Fat from fish, such as salmon, tuna, mackerel and sardines

Quick Reference Guide

Healthy Protein Choices For Your Child

Although we all know the standard protein choices that come from animals, many parents say, "My child doesn't like chicken and beef. What are some other protein foods I can give her?" Below is a list of foods that are a good source of protein and low in saturated fat:

Eggs	Beans	Canned Tuna and Fresh fish
Low fat Milk	Lentils	Pork Tenderloin
Cottage Cheese	Nuts	Chicken without skin
String Cheese	Tofu	Beef or Turkey Jerky
Greek Yogurt	Soy Nuts	Lean Grass-fed Beef

Healthy Carbohydrate Choices for your Child

Foods containing carbohydrate are plentiful in our diets, but some are healthier than others. We oftentimes think of only starchy foods as being a carbohydrate, but foods from other food groups can also contain carbohydrate. When choosing carbohydrates from the Bread/Grains group, whole grain sources are the best because of the vitamins and minerals they contain that are missing from refined (white flour) carbohydrate choices.

Fresh Fruit	Potatoes	Whole Wheat Bread
Dried Fruit	Quinoa	Oatmeal
Peas	Brown Rice	High Fiber cereals*
Beans	Wheat Berries	Low fat Milk or Soy Milk
Lentils	Whole Wheat Pasta	Yogurt

*Cereals w/ 3 grams of fiber or more

Quick Reference Guide

RESOURCES for Parents

Websites:
1. Nutrition Information for your family
   - www.kidseatright.org
   - www.choosemyplate.gov

2. Nutrition Action Healthletter, published by the Center for Science in the Public Interest (CSPI)
   - www.cspinet.org

3. Let's Move Campaign
   - www.letsmove.gov

4. Nutrition and Activity information for your family
   - www.energybalance101.com
   - www.fueluptoplay60.com
   - www.kidshealth.org

5. We Can! Ways to Enhance Children's Activity and Nutrition:
   - www.nhlbi.nih.gov/health/public/heart/obesity/wecan/

6. Fitness videos for Kids
   - www.fitnessbeginnings.com/exercise-videos.html
   - Fit Kids Fitness Workouts For Children - www.Amazon.com

7. *Portion Distortion II Interactive Quiz.* National Heart, Lung, and Blood Institute:
   - http://hin.nhlbi.nih.gov/portion/index.htm.

8. Academy of Nutrition and Dietetics for nutrition information and to find a Registered Dietitian in your area.
   - www.eatright.org

9. Medical and general health information
   - www.webmd.com

10. My blog and website for new information, add comments and share your stories
    - www.400Moms.com

Books:
1. *How to Get Your Kid to Eat…But Not Too Much* by Ellyn Satter

2. *Weight Watchers Eat! Move! Play! A Parent's Guide for Raising Healthy, Happy Kids* by Weight Watchers

3. *Your Child's Weight: Helping without Harming* by Ellyn Satter

Quick Reference Guide

RESOURCES for Kids

Books:

1. The Monster Health Book:
   A Guide to Eating Healthy, Being Active & Feeling Great for Monsters and Kids!
   By Edward Miller   (Ages 6-10)

2. Good Enough to Eat: A Kid's Guide to Food and Nutrition
   By Lizzy Rockwell (Ages 5-9)

3. Healthy Foods From A to Z
   By Stephanie Maze and Renee Comet

4. Fueling the Teen Machine
   By Ellen Shanley and Colleen Thompson (Ages 12-18)

Websites:

1. Body and Mind, Centers for Disease Control
   - www.bam.gov

2. General health
   - www.kidshealth.org

3. Healthy eating, activity, healthy body
   - www.kidnetic.com

4. Nutrition games
   - www.nutritionexplorations.org/kids.php
   - http://school.fueluptoplay60.com/tools/nutrition-education/games.php

Quick Reference Guide

About Jill West

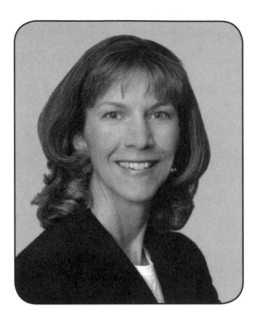

Jill West is an accomplished speaker, author, Registered Dietitian (RD), Certified Health Coach and Mom of 3 boys.

Jill graduated Magna Cum Laude from the University of Arizona with a Bachelor of Science degree in Nutrition and Dietetics and completed her internship at University of California, San Francisco.

For over 25 years Jill has worked with thousands of individuals and families as a Registered Dietitian, Nutrition Consultant and Health Coach. She has worked for several major hospitals including, University of California San Francisco Medical Center, Joslin Diabetes Center - an affiliate of Harvard Medical School and University of California Davis Medical Center.

Jill is a member of the Academy of Nutrition and Dietetics, the California Dietetic Association and the Diablo Valley Dietetic Association.